GROUP PROCESS
for the Health
Professions

THIRD EDITION

GROUP PROCESS
for the Health Professions
THIRD EDITION

Edward E. Sampson, Ph.D.

Professor of Psychology
California State University
Northridge, California

Marya Marthas, R.N., M.S., Ed.D.
Former Professor,
School of Nursing, Boston University and
San Francisco State University
Currently in private practice in Berkeley and Kentfield, California

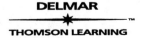

DELMAR

THOMSON LEARNING

Africa • Australia • Canada • Denmark • Japan • Mexico • New Zealand • Philippines
Puerto Rico • Singapore • Spain • United Kingdom • United States

Delmar Staff

Executive Editor: Barbara Ellen Norwitz
Developmental Editor: Marjorie A. Bruce
Production Manager: Gerry East
Project Supervisor: Marlene McHugh Pratt
Production Supervisor: Karen Seebald
Design Supervisor: Susan C. Mathews

Library of Congress Cataloging-in-Publication Data
Sampson, Edward E.
    Group process for the health professions/Edward E. Sampson,
Marya Marthas.—3rd. ed.
        p.   cm.
    Includes bibliographical references.
    Includes index.

    1. Medical personnel. 2. Small groups. 3. Medical personnel and
patient. I. Marthas, Marya. II. Title.
3. Interprofessional Relations.   4. Physician-Patient Relations   W.
62 S192g]
R727.5.S26   1990
302.3'02461—dc20
DNLM/DLC
for Library of Congress
                                        90-3906
                                        CIP

ISBN-13: 978-0-827-34352-8
ISBN-10: 0-827-34352-3

Table of Contents

v

Preface to the Third Edition

*T*here are usually three reasons for writing a new edition of an introductory textbook. First, new and exciting advances in empirical research compel authors to update their earlier works. Second, the field to which the text refers has been so significantly transformed that an updating of the previous work is required. Third, working with the previous editions in teaching contexts sometimes suggests that some materials need to be revised or recast.

Although we cannot claim that we are confronted with so many new and exciting empirical research findings in the area of group process that an updating on that basis alone is required, several significant advances have appeared recently. We have included these advances in this third edition. For example, we have provided a new chapter on Intergroup Relations (Chapter 9) and a new chapter on Negotiation (Chapter 10). These reflect new focal points of interest in the area of group process that are especially important to those working within the health professions.

It is clear to everyone both within and outside of the health-care industry that the entire health-care system has undergone very dramatic changes since the last edition of our text appeared. These major transformations demand that we take a new look at the role and functions of group process in the rapidly changing work life of the health professional. In order to reflect this transformed environment, we have significantly revised our opening chapter (Chapter 1) and prepared an entirely new chapter (Chapter 2) designed to lay a foundation for understanding the new demands for group process in the health professions. In addition, we have carefully reviewed all of the earlier material, updating our examples and recasting some of our approaches in light of these dramatic changes confronting the health professional.

Finally, working with the previous editions has led us to revise and refocus some of the materials presented in Unit II (examining the major characteristics of groups) and Unit III (focusing on theoretical perspectives), while incorporating only minor changes in the already strong and effective practical focus of Unit IV (addressing techniques of observation, leadership, and intervention skills).

The times in which we live and the careers that we pursue increasingly demand that we learn how to work successfully in groups. It has been our goal to add to the repertoire of the practicing health professional the knowledge and skills required to work effectively with groups, as both a leader and a member.

E.E.S.
M.M.

I

The Health Professional
and Group Process

*U*nit I introduces the student to the importance of acquiring knowledge and skills about group process by health professionals in order to improve the effectiveness of their daily practices. Chapter 1 introduces eight key functions that groups, both personal and professional, serve in all of our lives. A review of these functions demonstrates the centrality of groups to much of what we do. With so much of our lives involved in some form of group process, it makes sense to become more sensitive to how groups function and how we might function more effectively in groups.

Chapter 2 examines the dramatic transformations that have taken place in the health-care system during the decade of the 1980s—changes that will intensify during the decade that moves us into the new century. We argue that these changes increasingly have brought groups into the central arena of health-care practice, thereby adding the skills and knowledge of group process to the required repertoire of all health-care professionals who would remain current in their profession.

1

The Functions of Groups in Human Life and Health-Care Practice

*H*uman beings are complex creatures. We are *biological* organisms possessing qualities shared with all living systems and with others of our species. We are *psychological* beings with distinctly human capabilities for thought, feeling, and action. We are also *social* beings, who function as part of the complex webs that link us with other people. It is difficult to think of any activity in which we are not involved with groups of people. The range of activities in the health-care profession itself is broad and includes simple conversations with patients and colleagues, committee meetings, case conferences, hospital rounds, training sessions, and work with families and groups of patients. When we leave work for home, we become involved in another web of connections and interconnections: our immediate and extended families; friends; and members of our community. Even as our biological side is an ever present aspect of our everyday life and as our psychological character is involved in everything we do, so too are we, inescapably, participants in collective life as members of groups.

EIGHT FUNCTIONS OF GROUPS

To help us better understand this collective side of our everyday lives, it will be helpful to look at a map of the territory of group process. We will not mark this map with place names, however, but with eight group functions. Figure 1-1 summarizes these eight functions.

Keep three points in mind while reviewing these functions. First, any one group may and usually does serve more than one function. Thus, socialization and support are often found in the same kinds of groups. Second, any one group may serve different functions for different members of the group. For one member, the group may be a source of support and camaraderie, while for another, the group's primary function may be informational. Third, because each function we have listed seeks to define a central tendency or major emphasis, the meaning of one function may overlap that of another. We will now examine each function as it is relevant to the typical health professional's work life.

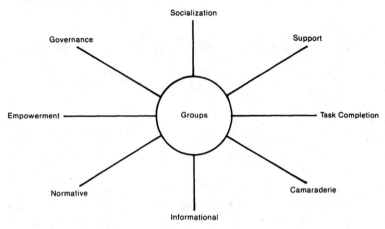

Figure 1-1. Eight functions of groups.

Function 1: Socialization

THE SOCIALIZATION FUNCTION OF GROUPS DEFINED: We are all born into groups and raised in the ways of our culture within groups. Throughout our lives, groups continue to serve the function of teaching and training us in the ways of our work and organizational culture.

There are three major topics involving the socialization function of groups that we will consider: (1) the role of primary groups in human growth and development; (2) professional socialization; (3) socialization into the culture of an organization.

The Role of Primary Groups in Human Growth and Development

The life history of human beings can be written in terms of the nature and types of groups in which they have been reared and in which they are involved over the course of their lives. We are all born helpless, unable to function or survive without the support and teaching provided by others. Contrary to popular, cynical myth, it is virtually impossible for any one to live independently of society.

The Primary Group

C. H. Cooley (1909) recognized early the critical role that *primary groups* play in the emergence of social feelings in civilized persons. For Cooley, a primary group involved close face-to-face associations of the sort found in the family, in play groups, in neighborhoods, and in informal work groups. Such groups are characterized by their sense of "we" and "our" rather than the individualistic "I" and "mine." These primary groups are the source of an individual's sense of self and remain vital sources to sustain that basic sense.

Hospitalism

Research discloses some of the serious consequences that face developing children who do not receive the kind of human interaction and contact that is typical within the primary group. While some criticism has been leveled at the findings of Spitz (1945) regarding what he calls *hospitalism,* his work stands as an important testimonial to the critical function that early group experiences play in our lives. Spitz observed children in institutions; although they did not lack physical comforts, they lacked the vital social stimulation of other human beings. According to Spitz, as compared with children reared in a more socially involved environment, these children not only developed lesser intelligence but also, as they grew older, were unresponsive to and disinterested in other people.

Bowlby's work (1969, 1973) adds further to this picture, demonstrating that a child not provided with strong attachments to a mothering figure tends to have difficulty later in forming attachments to others. It would seem, then, that one function of groups, especially those encountered early in our lives, is to socialize us into the ways of our culture, and as both Spitz and Bowlby suggest, to give us the basic qualities of humanity that are required if we and our civilization are to continue.

Although he worked with monkeys rather than human children, Harlow (1962) reached a similar conclusion: Unless the young monkeys grew in the presence of parents to care for them and peers with whom to play, they had difficulty later in developing heterosexual relationships and taking on parental functions vis-à-vis their own offspring.

Professional Socialization

When we think of socialization, we commonly think of just those matters covered in the preceding section on the primary group. That is, we tend to assume that socialization is something that is completed early in our lives; we believe that once we are socialized, the process has been concluded. Socialization, however, is a continuing event, never completed and always ongoing in our lives. Consider what happens to the newcomer.

We are all newcomers at various times in our lives: when we transfer from one unit to another within the same organization; when we change jobs; when we move from one community to another; when we learn a new technique, gain additional knowledge and skill; and so forth. Needless to say, if there are newcomers, there are also oldtimers. Most of us have been, and will once again be, in both positions within our job setting, community, or group.

As newcomers, we are in the position of those to be socialized: the ones who must learn the new skills and techniques, acquire the new knowledge, learn the ways by which this new community, organization or group operates. As oldtimers, we are the agents of socialization: those who must help socialize the newcomer, teach them the new techniques, help them learn the new knowledge, assist them in taking on the ways that our community, organization, or group operates—our rules of the game.

If we ignore the realities of ongoing socialization, we may not realize the socialization that occurs nearly every day in an individual's work life. We may also not be aware of the potentially stressful quality of socialization, especially for the newcomer. It is generally agreed that socialization is a stressful process (Nelson, 1987), presenting the individual with a variety of tasks, roles, and interpersonal demands. The manner in which a group helps socialize its newcomers, and the role of the oldtimers in this process, is thereby an important, but often overlooked area of group process. This entire issue has become increasingly important with the variety of organizational mergers that have taken place in the health-care system.

Group and Organizational Culture Under Mergers

As we will see in somewhat greater detail in Chapter 2, one of the characteristics of the recent health-care revolution has been the growing corporatization of the entire health-care system: that is, the increased presence of the large corporation that owns and manages a chain of hospitals and ancillary health services. One of the primary techniques through which corporations have grown so extensively in the 1980s has been through mergers in which one large fish (the parent corporation) consumes several smaller fish. Any merger of this sort joins together different group and organizational cultures into, at times, a jarring mix.

When we refer to an organization's culture, we include both objective and subjective elements. The former involve the different ways in which organizations arrange their physical work environments—including work areas, leisure areas, executive headquarters, parking facilities and so forth; the latter focus on ideas, customs and beliefs that characterize every group and organizational culture. Some organizational cultures, for example, are rather stiff and formal: staff are required to dress in particular ways; people are expected to address each other in a formal manner by using titles and last names; special areas are reserved for those with higher rank, and so forth. Other organizational cultures may be considerably less formal.

A merger of two organizations may bring together divergent cultures (Buono, Bowditch & Lewis, 1985; Kilmann, 1985). Unless careful attention is paid to the socialization issues of "acculturation" that are involved, the merger will not only go poorly on the organizational level (e.g., negative consequences for the organization's effectiveness in providing services) but will also produce high stress for the individuals involved. A merger usually joins one dominant corporate culture (this is the acquiring group) with a less dominant one (the acquired group). Thus, the pressure on the less dominant group to adopt the new ways of the parent culture can become intense, even disruptive, unless the merger is understood to involve socialization, thus requiring a period of time to plan and implement.

One investigation (Buono, Bowditch & Lewis, 1985), for example, identified several stages observed during the merger process. In the first stage, the less dominant organization experienced the take-over as though an invading army were entering to rule its territory. During this phase, there was a great deal of negative stereotyping and hostility toward the "invaders," and great concern expressed over the losses that the less powerful organization anticipated it would incur (e.g., loss of privileges; loss of personnel; loss of its own traditions and ways of doing the job).

The second phase identified by Buono and his colleagues involved a period of negotiation between members of the more and less dominant organizations. Members from each group sought to carve out a safe, familiar niche for themselves in the newly constituted entity. Phase three involved a growing sense of betrayal and desertion among some members of the less dominant group. They felt that some of their members had fared better in the new organization than others—including themselves—and so felt betrayed by their own colleagues. In the final phase, a kind of adaptation was noted, often helped along by major transfers of personnel or voluntary departures.

Function 2: Support

THE SUPPORT FUNCTION OF GROUPS DEFINED: Groups serve as vital sources of social support for their members, a source of collegiality and a place to turn when in need; in this, they often contribute significantly to an individual's well-being.

There are four main areas involving support that we will consider: (1) health maintenance and the supportive function of groups; (2) problem-related, self-help support groups; (3) the therapeutic milieu; (4) collegial support and professional burnout.

Health Maintenance and the Supportive Function of Groups

There is no longer any doubt about the vital role that groups play in health maintenance. Brownell & Shumaker (1984; Shumaker & Brownell, 1985) review much of the literature dealing with this subject. Some cynics behave as though they felt that their lives would be significantly improved if they could cease to interact with other people. The truth, however, is that without our connections to others, we become vulnerable to a variety of illnesses, both physical and psychological (e.g., depression), and our recovery is impeded.

An early study reported by Litwak and Szelenyi (1969) asked people to whom they would turn for help if they were suffering from various kinds of problems, such as a stomach ache, an appendectomy, or a broken leg. Their data suggested the importance of friendship networks in dealing with these kinds of problems. Even in the modern world, where fragmented and often superficial relationships predominate, groups of friends serve important supportive functions in times of need.

More recent work (Dunkel-Schetter, 1984; Vachon & Stylianos, 1988) adds to this picture in showing the important role that health professionals serve over and above family and friendship networks in providing social support. Dunkel-Schetter's (1984) study of the effects of social support for cancer patients, found that support was not only generally beneficial to the patients' adjustment to the stress of the disease and its treatment, but also that health providers (e.g., physicians and nurses) were mentioned almost as often as family members as major sources of support: in fact, family members were mentioned 34 percent of the time as major sources of support while health professionals were mentioned 30 percent of the time. In this study, friends received mention only 16 percent of the time.

Furthermore, when asked about the kind of support that proved to be most helpful, findings indicated that "health-care providers are seen as most effective when they provide a combination of direct assistance, advice or guidance, and emotional support" (p. 89). The investigator commented on the important supportive service that health professionals can uniquely provide: they have information that patients need to help them throughout their treatment, and the caring attitude of the health professionals includes the vital emotional element that transforms patients from mere receivers of technical aid to fellow human beings.

In many illnesses, social support tends to function in a rather complex way. In some cases, for example, friends and family members may actually prove to be less helpful sources of support than caring professionals. Attachments to the patients that friends and family members have may interfere with their ability to provide the kind of support the patient requires. Vachon and Stylianos's (1988) study of bereavement provides a helpful perspective on the complexity of the support process. Focusing on women whose spouses had just died, it examined the *density* of the widows' support network and its effect on their ability to cope with stress associated with bereavement.

Density refers to the degree to which members within a person's friendship and family network know one another. A highly dense support network is one in which there is a great deal of contact among the members of the network; in a low density network, one member has little contact with another. Vachon and Stylianos's research indicated that high-density networks, in which family members and friends were in close contact with one another, actually promoted less healthful conditions for the widows (e.g., more symptoms of bereavement, negative impact on her self-esteem, more disorders of mood) than did the low-density networks.

The authors reasoned that the widow must begin to learn new social roles that are consonant with her changed status in life, that these learnings are facilitated more by a low- than a high-density network. The members of the high-density networks were so overly attuned—not only to the pain of the widow, but also to the sharing of that pain among themselves—that they were unable to be supportive of the widow's need to begin to make the transition toward her new status. Similar effects seem likely for a variety of other kinds of illness and stressful situations complicating the otherwise neat picture portraying the positive benefits of social support on health. These data also highlight the important supportive role that the health professional can provide to the patient that members of the patient's family· and friendship-network may be unable to.

Mechanisms

Although the mechanisms linking social support to health remain unclear, study after study demonstrates a strong positive correlation between social support and well-being (Berkman & Syme, 1979; Cobb, 1976; Cohen & Willis, 1985; Jemmott & Magloire, 1988; Wortman, 1984). In the typical study, social support is defined by the number of personal and interpersonal resources an individual has. Someone with a high level of social support would have many friends and many attachments with others; someone low in support would be relatively isolated, with membership in relatively few groups. Well-being is usually defined negatively—by the person's suscepti-bility to a variety of psychological and physical disorders, including depres-sion, excessive sensitivity to stress, cancer, respiratory disease and even problems of the immune system.

Investigators (Jemmott & Magloire, 1988) have explored the relationship between social support and immunological functioning. It has been suggested that people with many group memberships enjoy better health as a result of these varied social contacts.

One issue that continues to puzzle investigators is whether social sup-port operates directly or indirectly. Evidence has been presented that sup-ports the indirect effects, termed *the buffering hypothesis* (Cohen & Willis, 1985). In this view, social support operates like a buffer that protects people when stress becomes too great. In effect, "People who have more adequate social support may experience less depression and anxiety and smaller increases in corticosteroids and catecholamines . . . when threatened by stressful events . . . ." (Jemmott & Magloire, 1988, p. 808). Those searching for more direct connections, on the other hand, have argued that whether individuals are under stress or not, social support has a broad beneficial effect on their health. Clearly, social support serves a vital function in human well-being and is one major function that group membership can play.

Problem-related, Self-help Support Groups

A recent edition of our local paper, in a section entitled, "You Are Not Alone" listed some of the following support groups meeting during a given week:

—Adult children of aging parents, offered by the community hospital, with group meetings to discuss resources available to family members caring for elderly parents.

—AIDS network, holding weekly support groups for people with AIDS; also, separate group meetings for the family and friends of those with AIDS.

—Anorexia/Bulimia, a weekly support group for patients as well as family and friends of persons with severe eating disorders.

—Attitudinal health for young adults, a peer support group for young adults dealing with life-threatening illness or serious accidents.

—Candida and chronic fatigue, with group discussions, support, and information about candidiasis, PMS, thyroiditis, T-cell abnormality, hypersensitivity, chronic fatigue, and related health problems.

—Cardiac rehabilitation, with a lecture for patients, family, and friends followed by group discussions.

—Teen drug and alcohol recovery, for teens, their parents, and anyone else interested in addictive problems for teenagers.

Clearly, self-help support groups of these sorts, with and without professional direction, have increasingly come to dot the landscape of most American communities, offering information and support to patients, their families, and friends, about a wide variety of health issues. While these groups have become a part of our health-care environment, questions continue to be asked about their usefulness.

Hinrichsen, Revenson, and Shinn (1985) report the results of a study of one such self-help group established for scoliosis patients. They examined members' reported satisfaction with their group as well as a variety of what the investigators termed "psychosocial outcomes": psychosomatic symptoms, self-esteem, mastery, positive outlook, feelings of shame, body image, sense of attractiveness, and so forth. Their data indicated that in spite of members' reporting being highly satisfied with their group, "there were few differences between club members and the comparison samples on psychosocial outcomes" (p. 77). This somewhat discouraging finding held for the younger patient groups; adult groups seemed to fare better on the psychosocial outcome measures, suggesting that support groups may not be as beneficial for everyone—or that only some kinds of outcome may be benefited by membership in these kinds of group.

This conclusion conforms with the research reported in Videka's earlier study (1979) of Mended Hearts, a self-help group for adults with cardiac problems. Members tended to show little difference from nonmembers on a variety of psychosocial outcomes, suggesting little overall benefit from the group. However, those who had retired early showed better adaptation to their cardiac problems from attending the group session compared with those who had not yet retired.

Although research findings usually temper our enthusiasm by offering a more complex view of the role of problem-focused self-help support groups, it is clear that such groups are a dominant and growing feature of our world, and that a growing number of professionals and corporations are turning to such groups as a central part of their own programs.

The Therapeutic Milieu

The concept, therapeutic milieu, originally referred to as the therapeutic community, first emerged in the writings of Jones (1953) and was initially applied to psychiatric settings. The concept refers to the purposeful use of the entire community or setting (e.g., unit in a hospital) as an environment designed to improve the patient's overall functioning (also see Cumming and Cumming, 1962).

The idea of employing the entire setting to improve the patient's well-being calls our attention to several important features of every environment that need to be taken into consideration, from its physical or ecological arrangements (Moos, 1976; 1979; 1980) to the weekly use of group process via community meetings to provide healthful role modeling and to inculcate values in the patient population (Daniels & Rubing, 1968; also see Haber, Leach, Schudy & Sideleau, 1982).

In their discussion of the use of the therapeutic milieu in nursing care, Haber, et al. (1982), point out some of the important functions that the weekly community meetings serve. The meeting itself is held every week and includes all members of the particular setting, including professional staff, other staff members and all patients. Haber and her colleagues point out important functions that such meetings can serve: providing a setting in which specific problems, including problem patients, can be addressed and worked through; and a place where patients can begin to learn values and norms relevant to their returning back home, by dealing with the host of the administrative and housekeeping tasks that any "community" must confront.

Moos's work (1976; 1979; 1980) has tended to focus less on the group process side of the therapeutic milieu (e.g., the weekly community-wide meetings) than on the importance of the ecological setting. His concern is in discovering how the physical arrangements of the milieu can be arranged to improve the patient's well-being. In some of his work with long-term care facilities for the elderly, for example (see Moos, 1980 for a brief review), Moos has examined such features of the setting as the following: the presence of hotplates or coffee makers in individual rooms; norms that permit residents to move and arrange their own furniture; rules allowing or forbidding residents to keep a pet (e.g., bird or goldfish); members' active involvement in setting residential home policies that affect their environment; occasions for residents to meet as members of a community. In general, his work suggests the important role that these and other ecological features of the milieu play in creating a healthful climate for living. Similar considerations can, and do, play an important role in most health-care settings, even though the properties of the milieu and its role in promoting patient well-being are often ignored.

A properly designed milieu will serve a wide variety of functions for patients and for staff. The socialization function is primary in many milieux in which patients relearn patterns of behavior that may have been lost through illness, and which are needed to function effectively back home. The socialization function is also apparent in the important role that community meetings play in inculcating values and ideals; and, as Moos's work reminds us, even the ecological setting of the milieu can communicate values (e.g., of independent living) if properly structured.

In addition, however, the milieu serves an important supportive function for patients and for staff. The community meetings provide an occasion where issues can be worked out and where support can be offered. Many of the other functions of groups that we will consider in the sections that follow can be incorporated into the functioning of a therapeutic milieu.

Collegial Support and Burnout

Another important supportive function served by groups is their role in helping professionals manage the many difficult situations they encounter on their jobs without succumbing to stress and burning out. Collegial support does not simply refer to being friendly to one's co-workers; it also refers to the very important role that collegial support groups play in helping people avoid burnout and its several job-related consequences. These include absenteeism, lateness, lack of commitment, boredom, cynicism, poor work attitude, poor work behavior, and a host of psychological and physical problems: undue fatigue, sluggishness, problems in thinking clearly and in getting jobs organized and completed, psychosomatic symptoms and so forth.

Health workers and those working during times of crisis are especially prone to stress-related burnout—perhaps because their work places them in so many situations in which others are vulnerable and in which the tendency to identify with vulnerable people increases the caretaker's own vulnerability; because the clients and patients often seem ungrateful or overly demanding; or because they work in an environment that is hostile, impersonal and uncaring (see Maslach, 1978; Mitchell, 1985). Many reasons contribute to burnout. Whatever the multiple causes, collegial support groups can serve a useful function in preventing burnout, in spotting its early warning signs, and in providing the kind of supportive atmosphere that will help people deal with stress.

Mitchell (1985) lists ten interventions that have been found to be helpful in mitigating the stress that many health-care professionals confront. Each of these has been employed in a structured collegial support group setting.

1. Use the group as a place and an occasion to vent intense emotions that people often experience, especially when their jobs place them in contact with patients and families suffering severe trauma.

2. Provide support for the professional, especially during times of high pressure, when stress is likely to burn out even the most stalwart of individuals.

3. Explore the meaning to the individual of various events. What a disaster means to those who must work with its victims, for example, or what working with dying patients represents to the professional health-care worker.

4. Help initiate the grief process that professionals may experience, but deny.

5. Use the sharing that takes place in a group setting to dispel the myth held by many, that they alone are experiencing the stress of the work situation so intensely. Knowing that one is not alone in one's reactions to a stressful job can help reduce that stress.

6. Reassure people that the intense emotions they are feeling are normal, not pathological signs of weakness or lack of professional distance.

7. Work with stress and burnout, charting a series of sessions covering the next several months.

8. Educate people, including health professionals, about the normal symptoms of stress and burnout so they will better understand what they may be experiencing.

9. Explain normal and abnormal responses to stress in their particular work environment, so they will better understand their own response patterns. Note that feelings of fatigue, problems with thinking clearly, general disorganization and sluggishness may be early warning signs of excessive stress and potential burnout.

10. Use the group as an ongoing resource of continued support and assistance.

A recent study (Leiter, 1988) provides insight into the role of collegial support in alleviating the effects of burnout. Data reveal that indications of greater burnout existed among human service workers who talked a great deal about their job but had few, if any, supportive relationships with their co-workers. The picture is relatively clear and supports the ten points noted previously: Co-workers can play an important role in providing focused support and helping people deal with stress and burnout before they become disabled by them.

Function 3: Task Completion

THE TASK COMPLETION FUNCTION OF GROUPS DEFINED: Most human activities require more than one person in order to be completed successfully; we join together and work with others so as to complete various tasks beyond the capacity of any one individual.

We will examine two aspects of task completion involving:

1. Specialization and the role of teams in professional practice.
2. The meaning and importance of cooperation in human task activities.

Specialization and the Role of Teams in Practice

Ours is an era in which most facets of everyday life, and particularly the area of health care, require specialization. The team has become the key unit of treatment (see Steiger, et al, 1960) in this time of comprehensive health care. Health professionals find themselves working closely with others representing different kinds of expertise in the care of patients.

A person's skills as a team member or organizer are vital to the effectiveness of practice. A team working with heart patients, for example, may consist of the physician, the cardiac nurse, occupational and physical therapists, social service workers, the dietician, and perhaps other specialists as well. Or a team working with colostomy patients may consist of a nurse specialist (teaches patients how to deal with a colostomy), a nutritionist (helps patients learn about proper foods), a physical therapist (helps patients rebuild strength and recover basic functions), a psychologist or psychiatric nurse (helps patients and families deal with the emotional aspects of the surgery), and perhaps even a patient advocate or social workers (to help deal with the variety of questions and problems that arise in connection with social services). Each person has different functions to carry out, but all share the same concern for the patient's well-being. But as we busy ourselves within our own specialized focus, it is all too easy to forget that the way the team works has serious implications for the patient.

Cooperation

The defining quality of a group is the interdependence among the members. Interdependence can be relatively low, as in an audience listening to a lecture, or relatively high, as with a surgical team, Also, some group members may be more independent and others more interdependent.

Interdependence, however, differs not only in degree but also in kind. Following the ideas proposed by Morton Deutsch (1953; 1962; 1969) we can distinguish between interdependence based on cooperation and interdependence based on competition. In a *purely* cooperative group, any one member's success or failure signifies success or failure for all the others. For example, if one member of a team does well, then the entire team benefits. By contrast, in a *purely* competitive group, any one member's success signifies failure (or much reduced success) for the others. If one person on the team does well, then none of the others can do well.

These two types describe two extremes of cooperation and competition. In the typical circumstance, these pure types are not encountered. In most groups, a mixture of cooperative and competitive interdependence exists.

Thus when the R.N. does her work well, not only does she benefit, but so too does the patient and the entire team with which she is associated.

It is important to recognize, however, that when we discuss interdependence as a critical defining property of a group, we do not thereby mean that groups can only be cooperative. Competitiveness is also a type of interdependence. If you and I are in competition, we must attend to one another's behaviors and adjust our own every bit as much as would be the case were ours a more cooperative situation. However, we would expect different outcomes for a cooperative as compared with a competitive type of interdependence. Research reported by Deutsch has suggested several important differences.

The Benefits of Cooperation

As compared with competition, cooperation results in

—*Greater coordination among members.* This is especially relevant when the group is composed of highly specialized members performing different tasks in which coordination is necessary for effective group performance. If such a group is more competitive than cooperative, individual members seek to do better than others, sacrificing the coordination of the whole group to their own desires to be on top and the best.

—*Greater division of tasks and specialization of functions.* This suggests that cooperation permits persons to specialize more, whereas competition threatens to undo specialization as members try to take on all the tasks for themselves.

—*Greater concern with and attentiveness to other group members.* Interestingly enough, although members of competitive groups are concerned with others' performances, in cooperative groups there is more genuine concern with others: all are in it together and so take more interest in others within their own group.

—*Better understanding of communication among group members.* Communication is rarely an easy matter; all the more important therefore to note that cooperation promotes greater mutual understanding than does competition.

—*Better quality of work.* Although we might have thought that competition within a group helps the quality of work, Deutsch's research suggests this is not the case; competition between different groups might help, but competition internally results in less effective work.

—*Greater sense of "we" and concern for the well-being of the group.* Cooperation promotes a truer sense of belonging to a group with shared goals than does the more splintering effect of competition.

—*Greater friendliness and feelings of self-esteem and esteem for the work of the group.* Cooperation again seems to facilitate individual members' feeling good about themselves and their work; competition may help the winner feel good, but seems to have some negative consequences for the self-esteem of those who do not reach the top.

Function 4: Camaraderie

THE CAMARADERIE FUNCTION DEFINED: The term, camaraderie, refers to comradely good will among friends. In serving this function, groups provide us those moments of joy, pleasure, and release that come from being with others.

It is self-evident that we find some of our best moments of joy in our interactions with others. The tensions of the day are relived as we meet informally in the coffee room with a few colleagues. We joke, we laugh, perhaps we cry. In any number of ways, we use groups to free ourselves from parts of ourselves that have been tightly contained in our work. Sometimes these are groups of co-workers; at other times, these are simply friends from other settings. Whatever the source, groups clearly serve an important camaraderie function. Therefore, do not seek to formalize or overly structure those brief moments of just being together joyfully with others.

Function 5: The Informational Function of Groups

THE INFORMATIONAL FUNCTION DEFINED: Groups provide us with a context for defining social reality, for setting performance goals and standards, for establishing priorities, for sharing our special knowledge.

Much of the knowledge we gain about the world in which we live—and the work we do in that world—comes from our associations with others in groups. We sit in a lecture hall or smaller meeting room to be taught about the latest infection control technique or learn the latest news about AIDS. In addition to these more obvious informational functions served by groups, there are several other aspects of the informational function, including (1) the important role that groups play in helping to form our attitudes and beliefs and in sustaining those attitudes and beliefs; and, (2) the role our group memberships play in defining the meaning of health and illness.

Group Definitions of Social Reality and Behavioral Control

Kurt Lewin's (1947a; 1947b; 1958) classical work is a key to understanding the important role that groups play in defining and anchoring our attitudes, beliefs, and behaviors; and thus, of the important role that groups play in both maintaining and changing these beliefs and behaviors. Although his initial efforts were concerned with changing eating habits by getting persons during wartime to serve less well-known cuts of meat (e.g., kidneys, brains, etc.), the issue remains the same, whether it is eating behavior, smoking behavior, or other health-related attitudes and actions that we need to understand or to change.

Lewin's analysis can be stated in terms of several key ideas:

1. Individual attitudes and habits do not exist in isolation but rather are related to the attitudes and habits of significant groups to which a person belongs or aspires to belong. The teenager, for example, may take up smoking as a habit because a peer group he or she belongs to or would like to join values smoking.

2. We tend to be rewarded with acceptance and a sense of sharing a common view of things when our behavior generally fits within the norms and guidelines of the groups to which we belong. We meet rejection, hostility, or pressure to change when our behavior strays too much from our groups' standards. A nurse working in a setting in which first names only are used is accepted as long as she or he generally follows this policy. Pressure to be like the others is brought to bear if this person breaks the implicit group understanding by using the more formal type of address (Dr. Jones).

3. Lewin suggested that since behaviors are frozen within supportive group settings, to change those behaviors it is necessary to *unfreeze* them from their setting. This means that the individual's support on the group in which the behavior is frozen must be reduced or the group's own standards (i.e., norms, guidelines, and implicit or explicit understandings) for the particular behavior must be altered. For example, the smoking teenager's habit may be frozen in a particular group of friends. That behavior can be changed if the teenager's dependence on the group is lessened or if the entire group's evaluation of smoking is changed.

4. To retain the new behavior the person must be within a group context that will support rather than undermine it. This involves a process that Lewin calls *refreezing*—i.e., locating the new behavior in a supportive group, a group whose standards enforce conformity to the new behavior. These ideas of Lewin have obvious relevance to such treatment programs as Alcoholic's Anonymous, to cite one important example. The member of AA both detaches himself from his former "drinking buddies" and simultaneously becomes a member of a group that opposes drinking.

Let us take another example that will help to clarify these points. Suppose that the issue involves helping a person to stop smoking or at a minimum to cut down significantly. First, we must recognize that smoking is a habit that not only developed within a group context but is maintained as a habit within a group context. Thus, to change the individual's smoking behavior we must work not only on the person but also on the groups that support that habit. For example, it should be easier to get people to stop smoking if we can bring them and other smokers together in the group to discuss smoking and perhaps collectively agree to reduce it, than by trying to deal with each individual alone. To deal with habits in isolation from the groups to which they are related is not likely to result in change; the person can return to the old ways too easily. Most self-help groups work along these lines. Thus to understand or to change poor health habits or to reinforce positive habits, we must work on the level of the membership group(s) rather than on the individual in isolation. And to work on the level of groups requires that we learn group process skills.

It is not stretching the point to suggest that understanding this key function of group process in the change and maintenance of individual attitudes and behaviors is indispensable to our practice. The promotion and maintenance of health means that the health professional must become sensitive to these processes and capable of working with them effectively.

Group Definitions of Health and Illness

Because we all live and work within groups, we are always subject to their understanding of most facets of our lives, including group definitions of health and of illness. There is a definite collective dynamic, for example, involved in the knowledge and reporting of various symptoms. It is well known that ethnic groups vary in their reporting of symptoms (e.g., Clausen, 1963; Croog, 1961; Zola, 1966). Zola's study of Italian and Irish patients at the several clinics of Massachusetts General Hospital, for example, suggested different responses to pain (Irish tended to deny pain more than the Italians in this sample) and to the presentation of symptoms by the two groups.

It is also accepted that members of different ethnic groups vary in their willingness to function in the role of the sick person (Mechanic & Volkhart, 1960). There is evidence suggesting the importance of training patients in the role of patient so that they may better participate in their own recovery (e.g., Harm & Golden, 1961). Because serious illness makes most of us dependent—and for some groups there is nothing worse than admitting one's dependency—these group definitions intervene to affect the possibility for successful intervention.

Some additional examples have arisen recently among professionals working in communities with a heavy influx of Asian refugees (e.g., Ishisaka, Nguyen & Okimoto, 1985; Kinzie, 1985; Owan, 1985). The refugees' cultural definitions of psychological illness and its treatment do not correspond with standard psychological or psychiatric practice. Each group (i.e., culture) defines what is considered a symptom of illness, as well as the appropriate treatment. In some cultures, for example, illness shames the entire family, creating an expanded definition of "the patient."

Ishisaka, Nguyen, and Okimoto (1985) detail some of the issues that a health professional will encounter when dealing with such circumstances in their study of Indochinese refugees. They noted, for example, that because of differences between English and the languages of these refugees, many key symptoms were not identified, in spite of the presence of a translator. They also observed that family values and loyalty are held in high esteem in the Indochinese culture, therefore any hint by the health professional that the patient's problem might be a result of his or her family situation will not be received with pleasure. Furthermore, the refugees' belief in the benefits of Chinese medicine and their distrust of Western medical practices will contribute to problems of compliance—particularly when drugs produce side-effects that appear to violate the vital balance within their system. Numerous other examples of the impact of cultural group membership on the definitions of health, illness, and treatment appear in this body of research.

What we are describing is a key informational function served by the groups to which we or our patients belong: These groups, in effect, establish the definitions of health, illness, and the role of patient. Practitioners need to become sensitive to these kinds of group factors or find themselves battling more than the physiological aspects of the disease.

Function 6: The Normative Function

THE NORMATIVE FUNCTION DEFINED: All groups develop ways to enforce the definitions and standards they establish for us; ways in which our compliance is encouraged, and ways in which any deviations are discouraged.

The informational function of groups emphasizes the way in which our understanding of social reality is structured by the various groups to which we belong; by contrast, the normative function emphasizes the degree to which those groups try to ensure that their members adhere to those definitions, encouraging compliance and discouraging noncompliance. We have devoted an entire chapter (Chapter 5) to a discussion of norms. It should be noted, however, that a very important part of group process involves the ways in which groups enforce the normative standards they have imposed on their members.

Some norms are quite clear and have been formalized into the rules and procedures of any group or organization. When norms have been formalized it is typical to find a similar formalization of the punishments that will ensue for any deviation from these practices, as well as procedures for dealing with appeals if the norms and the punishments are applied in an arbitrary or capricious manner. Many group norms, however, are never formalized, nor are the sanctions for deviation codified. One either quickly learns the ropes or, in failing to learn what is and what is not appropriate, is ostracized. We will return in Chapter 5 to a further discussion of the important normative function that groups serve.

Function 7: Empowerment

THE EMPOWERMENT FUNCTION DEFINED:. When a single individual seeks
to take on the world in order to change it, she or he may have little success
without the organized involvement of others who are similarly situated.
Groups, thereby, serve important functions by empowering people and helping encourage change.

The United States has a highly individualistic culture, in which the
individual is the valued centerpiece of the whole enterprise (see Bellah, et
al., 1985; Hofstede, 1980; Sampson, 1977; 1988). Most of us have grown up
so thoroughly immersed in this culture that we are not sensitive to the idea
that there are other ways of being throughout the world (Heelas & Lock,
1981; Shweder & Bourne, 1982). One of the main consequences of this high
degree of cultural individualism is the tendency we and others have to self-
blame. Put simply, if something goes wrong, who is responsible? The
individual, of course. And why is this so? Because if individuals are the centerpiece of the culture, they make it work. If it fails, they are responsible for
that failure.

None of the preceding is to deny the tactics we all use to cover our errors,
to rationalize our failures, to maintain self-esteem when we are assaulted by
the various problems and difficulties we all confront (Greenwald, 1980; Taylor & Brown, 1988). Rather, we are noting a dominant cultural theme that
even accounts for the omnipresent need we all have to explain situations
that have not quite worked out properly. What does all of this have to do
with empowerment?

To the extent that we define our personal problems as being personal,
and therefore caused by the failure within ourselves, we are very likely to
try to seek a personal remedy, trying to change ourselves in some manner.
The concept of the empowerment function of groups offers a somewhat
different analysis of human difficulties. To borrow a phrase from C. Wright
Mills (1959), once personal troubles are seen to be collective issues, we are
at the edge of seeking a collective rather than individual solution.

For this transformation in perspective to occur, we must become aware
that we are not alone, that we share many of the same problems with others
who are similarly situated. We can thereby begin to alleviate our sense of
self-blame and move from helplessness to hopefulness. While we may consider our troubles on our jobs as due somehow to a failing within ourselves
and so become discouraged, angry and burned out, when we discover that
others in similar work situations are having the same troubles, we realize
they are simply problems in the working conditions we all share. The resolution, then, is not to change oneself—often not possible under onerous
conditions—but to join with others, to organize, and seek to change the onerous conditions we all face.

Function 8: Governance

THE GOVERNANCE FUNCTION OF GROUPS DEFINED: Groups are often actively engaged in making decisions and serving as the locus of governance within organizations.

As we will shortly see, one of the consequences of the health-care revolution has been the development of massive corporations throughout the health-care system as well as the creation of various independent practice associations containing physicians and various other health-care providers. In the large organizations as well as the relatively smaller but growing number of independent group practices, governance by committee is the norm.

It is no longer surprising to find group practices organized into multiprofessional committees, involving nurses, physicians, other health workers and office managers who meet regularly to review and make decisions together on a variety of issues involved in maintaining a practice. Likewise, larger hospitals are divided into various governance committees, with specific areas of responsibility. Each committee consists of representatives of the various segments of the hospital and meets on a regular basis to make decisions within its purview, make recommendations to other committees within the hospital structure and so forth. The role of groups in decision-making and governance introduces us to yet another central function that groups serve in our daily lives and careers as health professionals.

A Case Example

Families, Inc., is an independent medical family practice group that operates in a large metropolitan area. The founding partners consist of three physicians, one nurse practitioner and a business manager. Additionally, Families, Inc., includes two registered nurses, a clerical staff of three and a physician's assistant. The entire group meets on a monthly basis for the stated purpose of governance, information sharing, and task completion. In these meetings, all group members, partners, and other personnel have one vote; anyone can bring agenda items to the meeting. The expectation in this group is that expressive needs such as support and camaraderie will be integrated into the group process.

In the March meeting of this group, Dr. Jane Rose presented the current information from the Public Health Department on the ongoing local influenza epidemic. Judy Parker, the business manager, brought a problem of rescheduling that required a group decision. The new R.N., Dan Marks, was told about some of the eccentricities of the way this particular practice functioned as well as about group policies that he needed to learn. Dr. Mary Stevens talked about the pressures she was experiencing at work because of the recent birth of her baby, and the P.A., Pat Smith requested and received permission to incorporate a newly acquired skill into his office practice.

It is clear that this one-and-one-half hour meeting is designed to serve a wide variety of group functions: governance and management of a large medical practice is accomplished; information is transmitted; specific tasks are completed; socialization is achieved; group support is both asked for and given; and at least one member is directly empowered.

Many of these functions overlap. For example, while much of the meeting was focused on helping to socialize the new nurse, information was also given precisely by Dr. Rose, and much time was devoted to the processing of information. And, while all of this was taking place, Dr. Stevens, who is currently vulnerable to burn out because of her increased work schedule, was able to ventilate her frustrations about trying to juggle work and parenting. The group was able to hear of her difficulties and to share their similar experiences and thereby provide her with support. Support was also provided to the new nurse and the P.A. The attention this practice gives to its members' express needs provides an on-going sense of camaraderie that is valued by all members of the group.

Families, Inc. represents a well-run practice that completes tasks and provides information, makes complex business as well as medical and nursing decisions, yet is able to provide a supportive environment in which to work. Group progress and good feelings create a sense of empowerment that provides strength to the entire practice and increases the patients' satisfaction with the kinds of services they receive.

2

The Health-Care Revolution
and Group Process

The 1980s have witnessed a major transformation in the health-care system of the United States that has affected every citizen—health professional and patient alike. The changes that have taken place in the "medical-industrial complex" (Relman, 1980), have been referred to as the "health-care revolution" (Kiesler & Morton, 1988).

Pinpointing the causes of any revolution in society is rarely easy. We frequently oversimplify complex phenomena in the hopes of locating the one major cause of the change. Although many factors developed in the later part of the 1970s to contribute to the health-care revolution, most analysts agree that economics and national economic policy played the most significant roles.

> The root of this revolution has been the spiraling cost of health care in the United States. In 1965, when Medicare and Medicaid were established, the cost of national health care was $38 billion (6 percent of the gross national product (GNP). By 1982, it was $355 billion (nearly 11 percent of the GNP), and it is projected to rise to $750 billion (12 percent of the GNP) by 1990 (Kiesler & Morton, 1988, p. 993).

In order to appreciate the meaning of these figures, we need only compare the mid-1980s U.S. GNP figure of 11 percent with the Canadian health care cost, which was 8 percent of their GNP, or the British health care cost, which was 6 percent of their GNP (see Reinhardt, 1987; see also Starr, 1982).

The ramifications of this situation have been substantial, affecting nearly every aspect of health care in the United States. In general, however, commentators agree that there are three major areas in which the revolution is most apparent:

1. The new technologies of medical and nursing practice have created demands for greater specialty training and increasingly narrow bands of expertise; these have expanded the need for interdependent teamwork among specialists in order to provide the highest quality care.

2. Economic policies have made health care a potentially profitable business and cost-containment a pressing national issue. New forms of health-care organization have emerged to provide services and to monitor practices so as to contain skyrocketing costs. These changes have had major impacts on the health-care professional's everyday work life as well as on the experiences of nearly every patient.

3. New forms of group practice, new structures of organization, and new systems for managing and monitoring health-care practice have come into being. Issues involving intergroup relations and skills of negotiation have become a central part in the everyday work life of the typical health professional.

Even a cursory inspection of the preceding three areas in which major change has been observed will indicate why group process has become increasingly central to the everyday work life of the health professional. The new demands of the health-care system have compelled persons who once considered themselves to be independent practitioners—relating directly to their patients—to become members of interdependent teams.

This trend has led the majority of professionals to become involved in negotiating with other professionals and corporate management over issues of practice, cost-containment, and working conditions. The aging of the population, the emergence of long-term issues in health care (e.g., stroke recovery, cancer, AIDS), and a new understanding of the social psychological elements of health care have caused professionals to become increasingly sensitive to the importance of groups (e.g., families, friends, support networks) in the management and long-term care of patients. Efforts to prevent as well as to treat illnesses that appear to correlate with modern lifestyles have led to programs designed to encourage healthful living. Most of these programs are based on a variety of group techniques, prompting a growing number of health professionals to learn how to work effectively in and with groups.

In this chapter, we will explore some of the major consequences of this health-care revolution for group process, examining, in turn, each of the three major themes previously outlined.

THE NEW TECHNOLOGIES AND
SPECIALIZATION: THE TEAM COMES OF AGE

Two hundred years ago, health professionals relied on their own eyes, ears, and touch, coupled with the patient's account to make a diagnosis and decide on the most appropriate course of treatment. In the mid-1800s, technological advances, such as the development of the stethoscope, provided additional tools to facilitate diagnosis, and, over the course of the next century, the introduction of the x-ray, the electrocardiogram, and chemical and biological laboratory tests further intervened between the health professional's own sensory apparatus and the patient. Each advance in technology added more information of an increasingly specialized sort.

Recent advances on the scientific side of health care have introduced new technologies for diagnosis and treatment that place an even greater distance between the professional's sensory capabilities and the patient and require ever more highly trained personnel. CAT scans and MRIs and chemotherapy, radiation therapy, dialysis, and organ transplants are but a few of the modern diagnostic and treatment procedures now available to health professionals (see Starr, 1982, for a helpful review of many of these changes).

A familiarity with this growing body of specialized technology is important for all health professionals. A specialized division of labor, however, is required in order to work effectively as the technology demands expert skills. This kind of specialization introduces many questions about the appropriate care of patients.

A patient is a whole individual who lives in an often complexly interconnected social world including spouses, children, family and friends, and work. Providing that patient with proper care therefore demands that those who are skilled in one area be carefully integrated with other health professionals in a genuine team effort directed toward the whole patient. The team approach to health care, in its turn, demands effective knowledge of group process.

Rounds and case conferences are examples of the fundamental importance of the team approach. Here, experts familiar with different aspects of the patient's case come together to review the situation, consider alternatives, and come up with an appropriate treatment plan. While it might appear that no special expertise beyond good common sense is required to work effectively in these teams, the best outcomes actually occur primarily where the practitioners are sufficiently experienced in group process to know how to coordinate the specialized expertise existing within the team and how to integrate that diverse information into the best treatment plan.

Specialization has also brought about a variety of other important uses of teams. For example, a team consisting of a physician, a psychiatric nurse practitioner, and a dietician might work with anorexic patients, designing a program that will best treat their complex physiological-psychological-sociological disorder. Cooperation within teams of health-care specialists facilitates optimum patient care.

THE TRANSFORMED HEALTH-CARE ORGANIZATION

Whereas the early hospitals tended to be freestanding community institutions and physicians independent small businessmen rendering services on a fee-for-service basis, the current health-care system is characterized more and more by multi-institutional national and international corporate structures and contractual relationships with providers (Aday, 1987, p. 277).

A few figures will help to illustrate what is meant when we refer to the corporatization of the American health-care system. Corporate involvement in health care first emerged in the United States in about 1968; by 1975, corporate involvement had grown substantially: at that time, the for-profit sector owned or managed somewhat over 72,000 hospital beds. That figure had increased by 68 percent by 1981, with the for-profit sector managing over 121,000 hospital beds (Starr, 1982).

Through acquisitions and mergers, a handful of corporations became dominant, controlling some 75 percent of the total number of beds that existed in the for-profit sector. A process known as *vertical integration* has increasingly come to characterize current and likely future developments in this sector (see Kiesler & Morton, 1988; Starr, 1982). In vertical integration, through a process of acquisitions and mergers, a single corporate entity takes on the wide variety of functions that were once parts of separately owned and managed corporations (see Scott, 1981). The new health-care conglomerate may, for example, run several hospitals as well as manufacture hospital supplies and equipment, operate a pharmaceutical company, control a testing laboratory, own and operate several nursing homes, and even become involved in the insurance business (see Kiesler & Morton, 1988).

The corporatization of American health care reveals a clear trend towards the centralized administration and standardization of a significant number of hospitals. Planning, budget, and personnel matters all occur in a carefully standardized manner and are governed centrally at corporate headquarters rather than locally under the guidance of a local board of overseers.

The transformation of the American health-care system has been rapid and extensive, and is by no means over. The field has . . . been reshaped both by changes in the funding of health care and changes in the organizational behavior of the increasingly large players (sometimes referred to as the "Supermeds" or the "Exxons" of the health-care industry) . . . we see the widespread acceptance of managed health-care plans, with the inevitable consequences of increased managerial control and organizational complexity (Kiesler & Morton, 1988, p. 995).

During this period of major for-profit expansion into the health-care market, the nonprofit sector did not stand passively by. Although its growth was not as centralized as the for-profit sector's—for example, in 1981, the top three nonprofits operated less than one-tenth of the total number of beds available in the nonprofit sector—the nonprofits did enter into active competition with the for-profits for a share of the total health-care market (Starr, 1982).

Seeking to maintain their own viability in this highly competitive market, the nonprofits actively entered into developing and marketing a wide variety of profit-making ancillary services, including nursing homes, weight loss clinics, addiction programs and so forth. Organizationally, the nonprofits had to adopt the same kinds of business and managerial strategies that work so effectively in every other sector of society.

The Management of Health Care

The corporatization of the American health-care system has brought about a variety of changes in the way in which the system is organized and its practitioners function. For the physician, accustomed to setting fees and operating relatively autonomously, the process of corporatization has meant a loss of autonomy to the corporation, and increasingly, a loss of control over fees, as large cost-containment organizations have emerged to oversee more and more of the payment process (Aday, 1987; Kiesler & Morton, 1988; Kramon, 1989; Starr, 1982). Changes of an equally major sort have affected the work lives of nearly every health professional, including nurses, technicians and ancillary hospital employees. These changes have not all been negative for professionals or patients.

Aday's review (1987) of some of the relevant literature, for example, suggests that there is little evidence to support the claim that the growth of the large for-profit health-care corporations have led to poorer quality health care. On the other hand, the evidence does suggest that the process of corporatization has not increased the access to health care of previously underserved segments of the population, nor has it reduced costs (see Aday, 1987).

Whatever else it has done to the health-care system's ability to provide quality service to the whole population at minimal costs, the process of corporatization has brought management and management techniques gained in the context of business and industry squarely into the forefront of the health-care industry and made group process an increasingly central feature of the health professional's everyday work life. The use of participative approaches to decision-making is an especially important management technique building upon the use of group process. Increasingly, hospitals are organized into a variety of decision-making and problem-solving committees, built around the managerial ideal of active participation and consensual decision-making. In one study of a hospital's psychiatric unit, for example, the staff's satisfaction with their work environment was found to be related to the degree to which they participated in decision-making (O'Driscoll & Evans, 1988). On the other hand, Fiorelli's study (1988) of interdisciplinary clinical team meetings involving staff from audiology and speech, nursing, occupational therapy, psychology, social services, and several other departments in a large hospital, found that although participation in decision-making was the assumed ideal, most of the treatment decisions were still made autocratically by the physicians.

In spite of what Fiorelli found to be the reality in one hospital system, the managerial ideal of operating within committees and by means of participation in decision-making continues to dominate most health-care organizations. One hospital with which we are familiar—we will refer to it as Hospital A—for example, located in a large urban area, functions with a combination of standing committees, specifically task-focused committees and committees that involve supervision within each professional group. There are regular monthly meetings held between the nursing supervisor and the head nurses. With one or two exceptions, membership on each standing or task committee comes from all segments of the health professional spectrum including physicians, staff nurses, laboratory technicians, quality assurance personnel, top level management personnel and so forth.

One of the main standing committees in Hospital A is the Ethics Committee, which consists of physicians, staff nurses, nursing administration, hospital administration, representatives from the pharmacy, representatives from the laboratories, the quality assurance officer, and the risk management specialist.

This same hospital has also established several special task force committees involving representatives from nearly every segment of the health professional spectrum. There is a task force designated to deal with research, another with educational projects, and still another to deal with developing ways to work with the families of oncology patients.

In response to a sexual abuse incident, Hospital A also set up a special problem-solving committee to develop a sexual abuse policy for the hospital. The incident involved sexual abuse of the staff nurses by one or two patients. The nursing staff complained to the head nurse of its unit that a male patient was acting in a sexually abusive way towards them and they were unsure of how they should deal with this situation or what hospital policy was in this regard. This particular patient would attempt to fondle nurses whenever they came within his reach, would frequently speak to them in sexually explicit ways, would expose himself to them, and on several occasions, directly asked a nurse to masturbate him. The head nurse checked with her supervisor who called together a special task force comprising physicians, nurses, quality assurance, and risk management personnel to review this situation and to propose a policy designed to protect the nursing staff from such abuses.

Other Uses of Group Process Within the Organization

The use of management techniques gleaned from business and industry has come to the health-care system, increasing the use of groups and group techniques within the workplace, while other aspects of the health-care revolution have also brought group process to the forefront. Increasingly, whether in response to the business side of health care or in response to a changed conception of the role of social-psychological factors in health care, many corporately operated hospitals (both nonprofit and for-profit) have established a series of ancillary services for patients. These services have been built around a team of health professionals and group process for the patients or their families including weight-loss clinics, sports medicine clinics, addiction-treatment programs, eating disorder clinics, sexual abuse and family violence treatment centers and long-term care programs.

In the typical case, a team of health professionals will deal with groups of patients, the patient's families, or in many cases, with groups of individuals from different families who are in similar situations, such as parents of alcoholic children; children of alcoholic parents; spouses of stroke victims; families of young adults with AIDS; or children with parents who have Alzheimer's. It is clear that group process is critical to the team's internal operation and likewise to the entire program that is based upon the use of family groups, patient groups, or shared-fate support groups.

PROFESSIONAL RELATIONSHIPS: INTERGROUP DYNAMICS AND NEGOTIATION

Not surprisingly, the health-care revolution has influenced the third reason the health professional of today must understand group process. The relationships that now exist among professionals within the field and between professionals and managerial groups have become a central element of today's work life for the typical health professional. Intergroup relations and issues of negotiation thus have increased in importance as matters of central relevance.

Intergroup relations focus on the processes that occur between groups: between labor and management; between ethnic groups; or, in the cases of greatest relevance to our concerns, between health professionals representing different segments of the health-care spectrum.

Taylor and Moghaddam (1987) define intergroup relations as *"any aspect of human interaction that involves individuals perceiving themselves as members of a social category, or being perceived by others as belonging to a social category"* (p. 6). By social category, they are referring to anything that people use to mark or identify themselves and others. "Male" and "female" are social categories of particular relevance in most groups. Thus, labor and management; nurse and physician; aide and R.N.; lab technician and nurse; and business manager and professional staff are all examples of social categories involved in the intergroup relations that occur in the everyday work life of the health professional.

It should be clear from this definition that intergroup processes can occur within a committee consisting of persons who represent different health-care specialties, for whom the category they represent is a key feature in the way they perceive themselves and are perceived by others.

For example, we interviewed a nurse who represented the nursing staff on the hospital's Ethics Committee. She described the difficulty she faced in gaining the attention of other members of the committee, particularly the physician members. They not only dominated in sheer numbers, but also in terms of the traditional authority they assumed and which others granted to them. Although every member of the committee had one vote and thus there was in that sense, a formal equality, the refusal of the physicians to listen to or solicit opinions from nonphysician members and the complicity of the rest of the group, this nurse included, in permitting this condition to persist, undermined the meaningfulness of the equality of voting. This nurse eventually did gain a voice, but nevertheless continued to be defined throughout by her social category: a nurse talking with physicians in the hierarchy.

Intergroup relations also occur when separate groups come into contact, such as with the collective bargaining that occurs between labor and management. For example, should a nursing staff feel that it has lost its voice in decision-making, it may organize and confront the administration in order to negotiate a change in hospital policy.

Negotiation

Issues involving negotiation increase in importance in intergroup relations. This is not to say that negotiation is absent within groups sharing the same social category (e.g., within groups of nurses), but rather to emphasize the important role that negotiation plays among individuals representing different social categories with different interests.

In Hospital B, policy is established by a committee entirely comprised of physicians. Although business management can overrule this physicians' committee, the physicians essentially control policy. One particular policy proved troublesome to the nursing staff. The policy required the nurses to take the vital signs of every patient at four-hour intervals. Nursing staff complained that this was virtually impossible, that taking vital signs would be the only activity for which they would have time. They suggested that taking vital signs once every shift would work better from their perspective, and that, in a few special cases, more frequent monitoring would be possible.

A series of meetings attended by nurses, physicians and the hospital administration was held to try and resolve this conflict. The physicians spent most of the meeting time lecturing everyone about the importance of diurnal rhythms and their impact on vital signs; they said that this was the foundation for their policy. In their turn, the nursing staff sought to explain why they were opposed to this schedule, even though they were well aware of diurnal rhythms.

This situation clearly illustrates intergroup relations; it also illustrates the importance of negotiation. Nurses and physicians face off against each other as members of their respective groups. Each group has its own understanding of its needs, interests, and obligations. The only way in which a resolution can be reached, other than the use of the formal authority of the physician, would be through some process of negotiation. Unfortunately, in this case authority won out over negotiation, at least in the short term.

Now that we have a preliminary sense of what is meant by intergroup relations and the process of negotiation, we will continue our examination of the impact of the health-care revolution on the changing relationships among health professionals.

Group Practice Associations

As several commentators have noted, the 1980s have witnessed "the rapid aggregation of providers into preferred provider organizations (PPOs), health maintenance organizations (HMOs), independent practice associations (IPAs), and the like" (Kiesler & Morton, 1988, p. 995; also see Aday, 1987; Starr, 1982). This transformation in the organizational form in which providers carry out their practice—which most experts agree will effectively put the independent provider out of business within a few years—along with the massive health-care corporations we previously considered, highlight the changing relationships that exist among different groups of health professionals.

In Chapter 1, we presented an example of one such group practice, Families, Inc., which combines the talents of several physicians, several nurse practitioners, doctor's assistants, accountants, and clerical office staff into an entity in which weekly meetings and annual retreats have become a way of life. There are many other such examples and, while not all of them may be as group oriented as Families, Inc., it is clear that all such practices must deal with a changed set of relationships among the various parties involved in the practice.

The Impact of Cost-containment on Intergroup Relationships

In the last decade the economics of health care has emerged as one of the most pressing and troublesome issues facing the entire nation. One of the major consequences of the skyrocketing cost of health care has been a strong movement towards cost-containment that has led to the development of new kinds of corporations dedicated solely to monitoring health practices in order to keep costs down (Aday, 1987; Kramon, 1989; Kiesler & Morton, 1988). By 1988 a few cost-containment giants were involved in monitoring the health care of some 100 million Americans.

These companies monitor the kinds of health services that are provided to patients, comparing the practices of a given hospital or physician with national averages. They are also involved in the second-opinion business, required by more and more insurers before they will fund various inpatient procedures.

These cost-containment companies are also actively involved in judgments about various office and outpatient procedures. And, as cost-containment becomes an increasingly serious economic matter for employers and insurers, these companies have begun to get involved in the actual case management of seriously ill patients—for example, cancer and AIDS patients—of patients recovering from strokes, and of high-risk pregnancies (see Kramon, 1988). Let us look briefly at some of the monitoring techniques that these companies employ and then examine the implications of these kinds of changes on the relationships between health professionals.

In a typical case, a patient, insured through her employer-sponsored policy, receives a recommendation from her physician that a particular procedure requiring hospitalization is necessary. If the patient wants to receive full insurance policy reimbursement for that procedure, she must call a special telephone number that will put her in touch with a professional staff member of one of these cost-containment companies. Often, the patient will meet with a nurse who will review the case and make a recommendation to the insurance company about the necessity for the procedure and the appropriateness of the costs involved.

The nurse has the company's national data banks on medical procedures and national cost averages at her disposal, which she uses when making her evaluation on a particular case. By comparing the proposed procedure and costs with those found nationally, the nurse can determine whether the charges are in line with common practice and whether the procedure itself confirms to standards established by the cost-containment company, based on their review of national data.

Although the nurse working for the cost-containment company will usually discuss the matter with the patient's own physician—and may even confirm the physician's decision—the whole cost-containment movement has transformed the relationships that previously existed among health professionals and has also intruded upon the once-sacred territory of the private practitioner.

Cost-containment companies possess huge data banks containing national figures on nearly every aspect of health care. This information can be used to raise serious questions about the practice of a given individual. Those questions, in turn, can lead to that practitioner's being dropped from the insurance reimbursement roles, or, to a lesser extreme, to reform the individual's practice. The same data, however, can also be informative about less costly practitioners and less costly hospitals and so provide a cost-containment view of to whom and where to send patients for medical and nursing work.

Of course, it is not only individuals who come under the scrutiny of cost-containment companies. Kramon offers the example of one major cost-containment company's turning up an unusually high tonsillectomy rate among the employees of a particular Texas Company. Such a suddenly high rate seemed puzzling and so they investigated further. They found the hospital that was performing the procedure to be, in their words, a "tonsillectomy mill." Upon being informed that "Big Corporation" was watching, the hospital's practices in subsequent years changed. The tonsillectomy rate certainly fell sharply!

These examples clearly illustrate the point we have been making. As cost-containment becomes a vital issue in national health-care policies and as companies develop to monitor and manage the issues involved in such containment, roles, and relationships among health professionals will change, often in very dramatic ways.

CONCLUSION

This chapter has examined the consequences of the health-care revolution for group process in the health professions. We have argued that the impact of this revolution on three main areas—specialization, organization and professional relationships—has not only increased the relevance of group process in the everyday work life and practice of the health professional, but has also increased the need for all health professionals to become knowledgeable about and skilled in group process.

We cannot overemphasize the importance that the knowledge about group processes and the learning of the special skills needed to work effectively with groups can play in either facilitating or in thwarting the success of the health professional. Nor, can we over emphasize the frequently overlooked fact that we are discussing knowledge and skills that can be learned and employed in one's everyday practice, and that in many respects are as important as the technical mastery that currently dominates training.

II

Some Major Characteristics of Groups

*U*nit II is directed at helping the student begin to see, think, and understand in terms of group process rather than simply in terms of the individuals involved. This issue is confronted in Chapter 3, with the argument that our cultural blinders lead us to emphasize the individual when we try to explain human behavior and that overcoming this blind spot is essential to improving our understanding of much of what goes on in our everyday lives, both personal and professional.

Chapter 4 examines the various ways in which human relationships are structured, beginning with role structures and examining, in turn, the structures of communication, attraction, and power that describe all groups. Chapter 5 introduces the concept of group norms and explores the impacts of group norms on the behavior of those subject to their rule, while in Chapter 6, a developmental perspective to our examination of group process is discussed. We argue that even as individuals pass through various stages in their lives, so too can we consider groups to have stages. Each stage comprises key issues with which the group must deal, beginning with the moment of its inception as a group and moving to the point of its eventual termination. By examining some of the central characteristics and properties that groups have, we hope that this unit will help students learn to frame their understanding at the level of group process.

3

Levels of Understanding: The Individual and the Group

*I*n 1936, investigators Allport and Odbert counted the number of words in the dictionary that refer to something about individual personality—words such as shy, assertive, friendly, and so forth. They found over 18,000 terms describing these and other qualities of personality. It is no wonder, therefore, that when we try to understand the causes of someone's behavior we seem to attribute it to something personal about the individual rather than to their circumstances (Ross, 1977). In fact, the study of this attribution process—how we attribute the causes of events and actions—has become a central part of the field of social psychology (the work of Kelly, 1973, discusses one important approach). The relevance of this area of investigation is, for our present purposes, simply to remind us of our tendency to locate causes in the personality of the individual actor. In other words, we seem to seek our understanding of human behavior at the level of the individual.

If, for example, a colleague with whom we work seems to be a bit testy, ready at a moment's notice to snap impatiently at everyone in the unit— including patients, visitors, and co-workers—we attribute his or her testiness to something about his or her personality. In focusing so closely on what we assume to be enduring qualities of the individual, however, we may miss the role that factors in his or her environments, work or home, play in behavior. Testiness may be less a quality of personality than a response that anyone in his or her situation would have to a particularly stressful job.

This example demonstrates that we can view behavior on at least two different levels, that of the individual and that of the situation. Different levels are like viewing platforms on which we stand and see the world around us. Standing on one level, we look out upon a sea of individuals, we try to understand their behavior by learning more about those individuals: they are simply testy people, quick to anger, and so forth. From another level, we look out on a sea filled with situational pressures and stressors: The person is in a difficult situation; anyone in that situation would behave in the same way.

Behavior may be "caused" by a combination of factors, some of which lie within the individual's personality, some of which lie within their situation. Yet, too often we ignore this complexity as we quickly "blame" the individual for her actions, neglecting to examine them at another level.

It is important to begin to think in terms of levels of understanding and the different perspectives they offer, particularly when trying to understand group process. If we are in a group meeting and see only individuals gathered together, behaving as they do solely because of their individual personalities, we will miss most of the group process, having failed to see the meeting on the level of the group. Most of this book is devoted to helping the student acquire ways of seeing and thinking at the group level. In order to see on this group level, we will first need to acquire some familiarity with concepts such as group and group membership. These concepts will help us refocus our attention so that the group will emerge as an entity in its own right.

THE CONCEPT OF GROUP AND GROUP MEMBERSHIP

Although groups are ubiquitous, something that we all participate in all the time, just what are they, really? What characteristics are critical in defining the concept, group? A group refers to associations between two or more persons who are in some kind of *interdependent* relationship to one another. Interdependence is one of the key defining properties of groups as opposed to mere collectivities or aggregates of persons. The concept of interdependence calls our attention to the ways in which persons are *organized* together; it refers to a situation in which what one person does has effects on another person's behavior or perceptions. If people interact and communicate together, taking one another into account, modifying their own behavior in light of the behavior of others, then we would say that for all practical purposes they belong to a group.

It is helpful to differentiate between a group and a mere aggregate or collectivity of persons who may even share something in common: e.g., all have blue eyes, or all wear white uniforms. Of course, when that shared characteristic becomes relevant to the members' definitions of themselves and others, then we have the beginnings of a *group*. At that moment, people begin to take one another into account, to develop interdependencies and organization. Any shared characteristic could become the basis for group formation: e.g., skin color, sex, clothing, etc. Most of us can recall occasions on which wearing a particular type of clothing has readily identified us and others as members of the "same" group: e.g., as a nurse on the ward rather than as a patient or visitor.

We have said that interdependence is a major defining feature of a group as opposed to a collectivity of persons. Interdependence has two related meanings. First, it focuses on the degree to which persons are organized together so that they no longer act independently, but rather, act interdependently. In this regard, a group is similar to a *system*; it is composed of parts or elements (i.e., the individual members) who function together, who affect and are affected by one another. Second, interdependence refers to the *shared awareness* that persons have of belonging together. While it is possible for persons to be members of a group without awareness of this belongingness, in the usual circumstances, members have a sense of the boundaries of their group; thereby, they have some understanding and awareness about who belongs in and who is out. We return to this point in a later section of this chapter.

A good example of interdependence between two people involves the classic interaction established between Jane and Bob, a not so happily married couple (from Watzlawick et al., 1967). Jane tends to be demanding and to nag Bob; Bob's response to Jane's nagging is to clam up, to withdraw and sit back quietly. This really irks Jane, who then nags Bob even more intensely. In turn, Bob is driven to greater withdrawal. Bob and Jane are members of a small group called a *dyad* or two-person group; it is clearly characterized by its interdependence: Jane's behavior is linked to Bob's and Bob's is linked to Jane's. Each person's response is a function of the other's actions. It would not be stretching the point to say that they are so interdependent that their definition of who each is stands or falls with their mate's response.

INTERDEPENDENCE VS. INDEPENDENCE

As noted, interdependence can be usefully contrasted with independence. Two or more persons are independent when one person's actions have no effect on the others; that is, when they do not form a group or a system. Two small children playing side by side in a sandbox, each wrapped up in a private world of play, could be said to be relatively independent. Jones and Gerard (1967) offer us some examples that sharpen this distinction between independence and the interdependent functioning that describes a group.

Pseudocontingency

Two actors running through a script are only minimally interdependent; each follows the script and uses the other only as a source of cues for his own lines. Jones and Gerard refers to this as *pseudocontingency* because each person's behavior is barely contingent (i.e., influenced by or linked with) the other person's; it is an example of relative independence between the persons.

It is not only script-following actors, however, who engage in such pseudocontingent actions. To the extent that a person plays out a role either rigidly following its plan regardless of the other's responses or totally ignoring the other's responses, he or she may be said to be acting relatively independently. Thus, a true group does not exist. A nurse, for example, who has a technical routine to follow and insists on doing it regardless of the patient's protests, comments, or anxious responses, is acting in a pseudocontingent, relatively independent manner.

Asymmetry

A second relatively independent type of behavior that Jones and Gerard discuss is similar to this last example; they refer to it as *asymmetrically contingent interaction*. In this form, one person's behavior entirely ignores the other's, but the other person's is dependent on the first person's actions—i.e., the other is interdependent with the first. Thus, the nurse may carry out her technical work without any receptivity to the patient; the patient, however, may gauge his or her responses to those of the nurse. Asymmetry is involved in this case in that the nurse's behavior is independent of the patient's, but the patient's is interdependent with the nurse's. Although this type of interaction is not usual in most encounters, in addition to the example cited, it can also occur in various kinds of supervisory and leadership roles. In this case, the leader acts without much regard for the persons being led; they, however, act interdependently with the leader.

Mutuality

Jones and Gerard reserve the term *mutual contingency*, to refer to the more typical form of group interaction. This occurs as each person takes the other's actions into account in setting the course of his or her own actions. Thus there is a mutuality, a true interdependence, and as noted, the essence of a true group.

By now it should be clear that interdependence is not an all-or-none matter—that is, either exists or does not. Rather, it is better understood as a matter of degree. A team of health professionals working together with the common task of planning and providing a patient's health care, for example, is undoubtedly characterized by a much higher degree of interdependence than those same persons sitting in a lecture hall listening to a lecture given by a visiting specialist. Furthermore, as the distinction between types of contingency suggests, members within groups may vary in their own degree of interdependence with the other members of their group. Some may feel themselves more a part of a joint enterprise than others; these latter may experience themselves as fringe members who take little from the others and give little in return. Likewise, some may act with relative independence of the others in their group while others may be mutually contingent (interdependent) with the others.

Summary

Let us briefly summarize. A group may be said to exist whenever two or more persons share some kind of interdependent relationship with one another. This interdependence can be based on different things:

—A common task or purpose that has brought people together (e.g., patient care)
—An attribute shared in common (e.g., in a group in which there are three women and ten men, the women may see their sex as a critical defining characteristic for a subgroup of three within the larger group)
—A pattern of interaction established together (e.g., the nagging wife and the withdrawing husband)

While interdependence involves taking one another into account in the mutual give and take of interaction, adjusting my behavior to yours and vice versa, it is a quality that varies in degree. Some groups are characterized by more interdependence than others; some members are characterized by more interdependence than others.

A NOTE ON GROUP SIZE

Now that we have a definition of the concept of *group*, it will be helpful to examine the issue of group size. For example, we have said that a group exists if it contains *two or more* persons. Is there no lower or upper limit? Does size make a difference?

Surprisingly enough, this is by no means an easy question to answer. We do know that as size increases, so too do the possibilities for relationships among persons. A dyad permits a relationship with only one other; a triad, or three-person group, permits six relationships, the six combinations of the three persons. A group of four allows twenty-five possible relationships. By the time the size of the group reaches seven, there is the possibility for some 966 relationships to develop among the members (Hare, 1962).

Sociologist Georg Simmel (1902-03) developed the fascinating thesis that a distinctly new phenomenon emerges when the size of a group grows from a dyad to a triad. If one person leaves or threatens to leave a dyad, then we no longer have a group. The preservation of the thing known as a group depends on both parties' continued commitment to remain together. Once we get to a triad or to larger formations, however, the life of the group extends beyond that of any one of its members. If one person quits the triad, there nevertheless will remain a two-person group. It is in this sense, therefore, that groups larger than two can be said to have an existence that is more independent of any single member than in the case of a dyad. Simmel also noted that triads permit the formation of coalitions and power relationships of the sort that cannot exist in dyads. Clearly, two members in the triad can join in a coalition to win their position over that of the lone third member.

Others interested in the effects of sheer size have noted a tendency, but only that, for larger groups to produce lower member satisfaction (see Hare, 1962). There is also some indication that beyond a group size of seven, persons have difficulty in observing and evaluating individuals as such; beyond seven, persons tend to relate to others more as members of subgroups or as "those people over there who share the same idea." In other words, with increasing size, persons may relate to one another more as stereotypes or as categories of persons rather than as unique individuals.

Others have noted (Hare, 1952; 1962) that as the size of a group increases, the time available for members to participate decreases; it becomes more difficult for any one member to speak. In fact, only bolder and more aggressive members may speak as the size of a group increases; those who are generally quiet persons will often be left out of discussions in larger-sized groups. Greater size, however, also permits a greater number and a greater diversity of resources among the group members. With very small groups, composed of only two, three, or even four persons, there is little diversity possible. As size increases, however, the resources potentially available for problem solving increases.

Now, having noted that size apparently makes some difference, at least at the lower and upper limits (e.g., when too many people are present even to discuss matters), we would agree with Cartwright and Zander (1968), who suggest that the basic group processes involved are highly similar whatever the size, at least within the range of the typical small group: e.g., from two to fifteen persons. Indeed, a dyad may create more pressures on the two members to remain together lest there be no group; yet evidence suggests that similar pressures are brought to bear on members of even larger groups.

One can fruitfully speak of group process without attempting to provide any fine distinction between groups of two through groups of fifteen or so. Within the health professions, groups tend to be relatively small: the dyadic relationship with a patient or a colleague, the team-type relationship, the relationship with the family as a group, the relationship to patient groups or speciality-ward groups, and so forth. The student of group process should remain attentive to the possible effects of group size; however, we are suggesting that within a rather extensive range (e.g., two to fifteen), size may have less effect than other factors.

CHARACTERISTICS OF THE SOCIAL RELATIONSHIPS WITHIN GROUPS

Let us return to our discussion, from Chapter 1, of the contribution of Cooley, particularly his concept of a primary group; this will provide us with a further analysis of the social relationships within groups. Recall that Cooley introduced the concept of the primary group to refer to the relatively intimate, face-to-face association of persons who felt a strong sense of "we" a sense of camaraderie and of belongingness. This is the type of group relationship that characterizes the family, small friendship groups, and often small, informal groups in work settings. Primary-group relationships are based on close and informal ties that link persons together. The emphasis is on informality and closeness and on the satisfaction of personal needs.

By contrast, we find what can be called secondary or more formal group relationships. These, while often small in size and face to face, are not as intimate and close as primary relationships. Secondary or formal group relationships tend to be those we also encounter at work, when we occupy our work roles and relate to others as nurse to doctor, nurse to nurse, professor to student, health professional to patient. Formal and secondary group ties typically engage only a part of the totality that is us; we are mainly defined by our job and what we do. Secondary-group relationships tend to emphasize work and the accomplishment of some tasks; they emphasize greater rationality and impersonality. Primary or informal group ties encompass more of who we are, extending beyond our work roles and into our personal and often private selves.

All of us belong to both types of groups and experience both kinds of group relationship. Much of the work of health professionals involves the person in more formal, secondary-type groups and relationships. It is the job speciality that has brought persons together with others to form a group or a team. Yet even here more informal, primary-type relationships can and do evolve. Persons form smaller friendship groups within the formal workgroup setting.

The student of group process must be sensitive to these different types of group relationships and must develop a facility in working with both. For example, the nurse who is a member of a speciality team is involved in a formal group; yet that same nurse may then work with the patient's family, at which point she is working within a primary group, though not one in which she is a member. Furthermore, that nurse may have her own primary groups in other aspects of her job. Although the basic processes for both types of group relationships are similar, a sensitivity to this distinction can facilitate the work one does. It is usually considered poor practice, for example, to attempt to impose primary-group expectations of personal and more intimate exchange of feelings in a secondary or more formal group; likewise it is usually taken to be peculiar if one seeks to relate more formally within a primary group: e.g., by setting up strict rules of procedure for decision-making when primary-type groups tend to rely on more informal, personal bases for reaching their decisions.

The primary-secondary or informal-formal distinction in social relationships has been further refined by other analysts of group processes; they have noted primary-like and secondary-like functions in all groups, whether they be primary or secondary in their dominant form (e.g., Bales, 1955a, 1955b; 1958; 1970; Bion, 1959; Homans, 1950). For example, though a family is a primary group, serving personal needs for its members, it has functions to perform that have a secondary-like quality: e.g., working for a living in order to maintain the family; apportioning family tasks among the members; dealing with budgetary matters. Likewise, though the main concern of a work group (e.g., health professional team) may emphasize impersonality and formal distance between members so that its job can be done, it also must be concerned with the primary-like functions involving member's feelings about one another.

A useful way of focusing on this distinction within all groups is to speak about two types of functions that all groups must serve: task-related or instrumental functions and member-related, interpersonal functions, involving group maintenance. The former are similar to secondary relationships; the latter, to primary relationships. This distinction calls our attention to the two worlds of group process. The one world emphasizes external matters, such as getting the job done or the group's task completed; the other emphasizes internal matters; such as helping to maintain the group's morale and good feelings among the members. Many theorists have employed this same type of distinction:

—Bales speaks about task functions and socioemotional functions

—Homans has referred to a group's external system as contrasted with its internal system

—Bion speaks of a work group as distinct from an emotionality group

This is an important distinction, one which we will encounter again in several other contexts throughout this text. It informs us that even within highly formalized work groups, based almost entirely on secondary-type relationships (e.g., doctor to nurse; nurse to patient), primary-type issues are present. While the nurse may be relating to her patient in a rather formal manner, emphasizing her technical expertise, the effectiveness of her work hinges significantly on the patient's acceptance of her care plan. This acceptance depends on the ways in which the nurse has been able to deal with the more primary, informal aspects of her relationship to the patient.

Similarly, a team leader may have substantial expertise and technical know-how in his field and thereby be very skilled in dealing with the external or task functions of the team; yet the team may not function effectively as a team and his own expertise may not be translated into member acceptance because he has failed to deal adequately with internal issues of team maintenance.

The reverse of the preceding is also a realistic possibility. A team leader may emphasize internal matters of group maintenance to the exclusion of external, task-related issues. Thereby, she may have a team in which members have good feelings about one another and in which personal needs for more intimate, close relationships are met, but the team may nevertheless fail in its mission to get its job accomplished. Obviously, therefore, if two sets of function characterize all group processes, both must be adequately handled for effective group functioning. We return to this distinction again in a later section of this chapter.

GROUP MEMBERSHIP: WHO'S IN AND WHO'S OUT?

Who is *in* a group and who is *out*? Who is a member and who is a nonmember? Where does the boundary of the group extend? These are all critical issues of group membership. Membership in some groups, of course, may not appear to be an issue; everyone seems to know who is in and who is out. The more formal the group, the more its boundaries are defined by formal institutions and regulations: e.g., this is a classroom; this is a unit in the hospital. In such settings, the boundary issues may be less troublesome. But even here, membership issues crop up. For example, is the hospital director a member of this group or not? Are the patients on the unit members of the nursing team or not? Are doctors who attend rounds only on occasion members of this group or not? Are persons who hardly participate in the team's work really members or not?

But why is the membership or boundary issue important to understand? Basically, group membership lets us know who we expect to behave like a group member and who we do not expect to behave the way group members should. Being defined as a member of a group places people within the boundary of the system and sets up certain expectations for their behavior toward other members, others' behavior toward them, and members' behavior toward those outside the group. We do not expect nonmembers to act the same way that members are expected to act; we do not bring sanctions to bear on nonmembers for deviating from these expectations; nor do nonmembers expect to be sanctioned (i.e., rewarded or punished) for straying from the behavior expected of members. Therefore, membership indicates who is and who is not included within the power and influence sphere of a group.

Nonmembership

There have been several noteworthy efforts to help define group membership and especially nonmembership (Merton, 1957; Jackson, 1959). To understand membership and nonmembership, we must know two things: something about the group members and something about the nonmembers. The important element from the perspective of the group members involves what Jackson has termed *acceptance* and Merton, *eligibility*.

Eligibility

Acceptance or eligibility refers to the degree to which there exists a position in the group for a nonmember. We can speak of a dimension of eligibility. At one end, we have nonmembers who are defined as eligible for membership; for them acceptance is a real possibility. At the other end, we have nonmembers who are ineligible for membership, for whom negative acceptance (rejection) is the real possibility.

For example, nursing has specific degree requirements for its membership; persons who have the degree are eligible for membership in numerous groups within nursing, whereas persons without the proper degree are ineligible, at least until they obtain their degree. Until that time, they are excluded from membership. A group that actively excludes persons because of their age, their sex, their race, their religion, or similar characteristics is one that declares many types of persons to be ineligible for membership. Caste systems in India provide one such example, as do many kinds of professional and private associations in the United States. The family typically defines as ineligible for membership all those persons not linked by blood or by marriage into the group. If marriage across religious lines, for example, is not acceptable to a given family, then its boundaries extend to include as potential members only those of the same religion as existing family members. Intermarriage thereby fails to extend the group's boundaries; rather, both the blood kin and that person's spouse are rejected.

Attraction

The second element in our equation for understanding the issues of membership and nonmembership is derived from the nonmembers themselves. Jackson refers to this dimension as *attraction,* while for Merton it involves the nonmembers' *attitudes toward becoming a member.* Again, we have a dimension. One end represents positive attraction; the nonmember aspires to belong to the group. At the other end, we have negative attraction; the nonmember is actively motivated not to belong to the group.

When we apply the concept of attraction to actual group members rather than to nonmembers, we are dealing with the very important concept of *group cohesiveness.* Cohesiveness is based on an analysis of a groups' total profile with respect to members' attraction to the group. A group is said to be highly cohesive and thereby likely to function effectively insofar as all persons who are members are highly attracted to their group; low cohesiveness represents a condition in which members generally belong to the group but are not highly attracted to this membership. When we are dealing with nonmembers, however, the issue is not one of cohesiveness, but rather involves the nonmembers' attitudes toward becoming a member.

Table 3-1 provides a summary of *nonmember types* based on an analysis of the group's definition of a person's eligibility for membership and the nonmember's attraction toward joining the group. A plus (+) indicates positive eligibility or a positive attitude toward joining; a minus (−) indicates ineligibility or negative attraction.

Table 3-1 tells us several important things. The analysis suggests that nonmembership is a highly differentiated matter. The *in* vs. *out* issue, therefore, is more complex than we might otherwise have thought. There are various ways of being outside the boundaries of a group. But, even more significantly, these different ways of being outside have different implications for those who are inside: i.e., for the members. Antagonistic nonmembers may force a group toward internal cohesiveness almost as a defense against the hostility from outside. On the other hand, marginality is undoubtedly more painful for the nonmember than for the members; it describes a nonmember who would like to be a member but who is not eligible for such membership. Of course, it may have some appeal to a group because it can enable the members to feel very exclusive.

Table 3-1. Types of Nonmembers

	Eligibility	*Attraction to Join*
Candidate for membership	+	+
Autonomous nonmember	+	−
Marginal nonmember	−	+
Antagonistic nonmember	−	−

Marginality

The student of group process can benefit substantially from a knowledge of these types of nonmembers. For example, a marginal nonmember, as we have noted, is in an especially difficult, often disturbing position vis-à-vis a particular group. Marginal people crave acceptance but are not yet eligible and so really do not know where they stand in relation to others. This could describe the student nurse who is doing an internship at a hospital and is not yet fully accepted as a member of the professional staff. She is marginal and will typically reflect some of the symptoms of this marginality: e.g., high anxiety levels, confusion, excessive efforts to please or excessive rebellion, loneliness, anger, perhaps despair and depression. Knowing that a person is marginal to a group can not only help our diagnosis of some of that person's difficulties; it can also facilitate our intervention on his or her behalf. If we are the leader or organizer of the group, we can actively invite the marginal person in; even though the person is not, strictly speaking, eligible for full membership, he or she can be brought in and treated more as a member and less as a marginal person.

Groups we may deal with in practice (e.g., families and patient groups) may also have marginal nonmembers. It is not that unusual to find adolescents, for example, to be marginal within their own families. Technically they belong but psychologically they are not yet considered eligible for full adult status within the family. They are marginal and show many of the symptoms of their marginality. Again, the health professional working with this group can help undo the adolescents' marginality: e.g., working to include the adolescent in the family, helping the family explore the issue of marginality, and so forth.

The Candidate and the Autonomous Nonmember

Two further interesting cases of nonmembership involve those who are candidates and those who are autonomous.

A group that confronts many autonomous nonmembers—that is, those who are eligible for membership but who are not attracted to membership—finds itself in a difficult position. What must it mean for members to know that many eligibles do not wish to join? For example, what would the ANA or AMA be like if few of those eligible for membership actually became members? As Merton noted, "Rejection by eligibles symbolizes the relative weakness of the group by emphasizing its incompleteness of membership just as it symbolizes the relative dubiety of its norms and values that are not accepted by those to whom they should in principle apply" (1957, p. 291).

For example, a residency program in Family Practice gauges its own value by computing a matching score based on comparing the number of high-ranking applicants it accepts with the number who actually accept membership in the program. A high percentage indicates that the program is able to match well—that is, to attract those persons to join the group that it most wants to join. A low percentage, by contrast, signifies a basic weakness in the group; few of those it wants to join seek to join it; they go elsewhere. The morale of the members of the program is significantly affected by these percentages. The low-percentage match indicates, as Merton has noted, that something about the group's norms, values, and effectiveness is doubtful. Or, take another example.

> Teaching Team A at a school of nursing has a long-standing reputation as being high in conflict, a difficult group to work with. Each year the team must search for new members to complete its speciality teaching requirements. Many candidates are eligible to join the team; the faculty is large and there are additional openings for several new persons to be hired. However, literally none of those many who are eligible wants to join the team. Team A can be contrasted with Team B at the same school; all of the eligible candidates are eager to join Team B. Its reputation is of a better, more harmonious work group, one in which the person can function more effectively as a nurse-educator.

In terms of Table 3-1, Team A has many autonomous nonmembers, while Team B has many candidates for membership. The presence of so many autonomous nonmembers lowers the morale and potential effectiveness of Team A; the existence of many candidates, on the other hand, boosts the morale and effectiveness of Team B.

The importance of group morale for group effectiveness is rather apparent. What may not be as apparent, however, is the implication of this analysis of nonmembership for understanding one of the bases for high or low morale. The student of group process will benefit substantially from a recognition that *morale is affected by nonmembers as well as by members*. Diagnosing a morale issue, therefore, may require an understanding of who does *not* belong to the group. It is difficult for a group to maintain itself or to think well of itself if too many eligible members fail to join. The group's leader might do well to consider the implication of these nonmembers for group functioning.

REFERENCE GROUPS AND MEMBERSHIP GROUPS

The concept of a nonmember who is a candidate for membership, the person who is both positively attracted to membership in the group and is eligible for membership, introduces us to the important idea of *reference group* (see Hyman, 1942; Newcomb, 1943; 1958). When we speak of a reference group, we mean a group in which a person either may or may not have membership; in either case, it is a group the person uses as a reference source for his or her own attitudes, values, and behaviors.

There are three possibilities. First, a reference group may also be a membership group. This is a group the person belongs to, identifies with, and uses to guide his or her own points of view. Jackson refers to this as *psychological membership* in a group. Second, a person may be a member of a group, yet not consider it to be his or her reference group. Jackson refers to this person as a *rebellious member*. Although such people belong to the group, they are negatively attracted to it; they use other groups as the source of their own values and attitudes. For example, a person may be a member of a team and yet so dislike membership on that team that he adopts the values of another team as his own rather than his own team's values.

Finally, a person may not be a member of the group and yet be a candidate for membership; this person uses the group she is not yet in as a basis for her own attitudes, values, and behaviors. The process, termed *anticipatory socialization*, usually occurs under these circumstances. The nonmember candidate begins to act in the way that actual members act, adopting the members' mannerisms, clothing (if possible), values, and such. This is anticipatory socialization in that it helps prepare the candidate prior to membership for taking on the characteristics proper to actual membership. Thus, the person, anticipating membership, begins to become socialized into the ways of membership.

Nursing students in training will be eligible for membership in many groups in their field; their training may be seen as involving anticipatory socialization, by which process they begin to adopt the perspectives of those groups for which they are candidates for membership though not yet actual members. In this way, when they graduate and become actual members, they are already able to behave as members do.

The reference-group concept has proved very useful for understanding a variety of phenomena about human behavior. In addition to examining the effects of actual group membership on member behavior, the reference-group concept informs us that groups influence nonmembers who aspire to belong and are candidates for membership. Therefore, in understanding group process, we must expand our focus and examine both membership groups and nonmembership, reference groups.

The reference-group concept also helps us understand how persons resist being influenced or affected by their present membership groups. A student, for example, may reject her university as a reference group even though it is her membership group. She may successfully accomplish this by maintaining her family as her key reference group, retaining its attitudes and values rather than adopting, for example, the more liberal attitudes of her university membership group (Newcomb, 1958).

MEMBERSHIP ALTERNATIVES AND MEMBERSHIP TYPES

Thibaut and Kelley (1959) provide us with two further concepts that amplify our understanding of the process involved in group membership. These investigators make a distinction between a group member's *attraction* to the group and his or her *dependency* on the group. As we have discussed, a member's attraction refers to the degree to which that person likes or dislikes being in the group. Dependency, however, is a somewhat different dimension of membership. To be dependent on a group means not to have equally attractive alternative groups for membership. A member might be highly dependent on one particular group because there are no other groups that are more attractive or because the costs involved in leaving the group reduce the attractiveness of other possible alternatives.

For example, an R.N. may have to retain her employment in a given hospital in a community for family reasons. In a tight job market, she may have few alternative employment possibilities (i.e., few alternative group memberships) and so is highly dependent on her present group membership. Likewise, the costs involved in moving out of the community to find work and memberships elsewhere may be so great as to make any alternatives less attractive. By contrast, in a good job market or with a different family situation, mobility possibilities may be so great that dependency on any one group may be low; numerous alternatives help the R.N. feel relatively independent of any one membership.

A member's dependency on a group is a matter of degree; it can have important implications for how that member functions within the group and how the group as a whole functions. A member who feels minimally dependent on a group, having many equally attractive alternatives, for example, will be less influenced by the group than will a person who is more highly dependent; the latter is likely to go along with the group because no other choices are available. Obviously, resistance to group influence can be greater if people can simply pack up and leave than if that is the only group in town and they must stay. High dependence, of course, does not necessarily make for an effective work group; just the opposite possibility also exists. The burning resentment of those who have few alternatives often shows up in poor work performance, lateness, refusal to take responsibility for tasks that must be done, general apathy, nonparticipation, and so forth.

In the Thibaut and Kelley analysis, attraction and dependency can vary. Four possibilities can be represented:

	Attraction	*Dependency*
Type A	High	High
Type B	High	Low
Type C	Low	High
Type D	Low	Low

Type A describes the member who is attracted to the group and highly dependent on it; we would not expect great resistance or resentment in such a member. Although such people have few alternatives to their present group membership, they are highly satisfied with the situation. Type B describes people who are highly attracted to the group but not dependent on it; these members have alternatives and so are more able to resist undue group pressure; yet they need not resent this group, to which they are highly attracted. Type C describes people who are more highly dependent on the group than attracted to it. These are types of members who harbor much resentment; they are literally stuck in a setting that is not much to their liking. Type D describes what might best be termed apathetic group members who are neither very attracted to the group nor highly dependent on it; alternatives do exist, but they seem to remain in the group, showing neither enthusiasm nor resistance.

SUMMARY AND CONCLUSIONS

Chapter 3 suggested that we can adopt two very different levels of analysis in our efforts to understand group process: seeing what takes place from the level of the individual members of the group; and seeing what takes place from the level of the group as a special entity in its own right. We noted that most of us typically adopt the individualistic framework for our understanding and that the purpose of this chapter, and much of this book, is to help us begin to see from the level of group process.

In orienting us to "the group," this chapter examined the concepts of groups and of group membership. We noted how the concept "group" hinges importantly on the idea of interdependence, and that interdependence itself is a matter of degree and kind. Formal relationships, for example, provide a type of interdependence among people that differs from the types found in more informal associations among friends. In examining the concept of group membership, we observed several complex possibilities and reviewed some of the implications that various forms of membership *and* nonmembership have for the ongoing dynamics of a group.

4

Roles and the Structure of Groups

*I*n this chapter, we will examine several ways in which groups are structured. Before we can consider the structures one typically finds within a group, however, we must first examine the concept of structure. This will give us still another set of tools—the concepts of groups and group membership were the first—with which to examine group process from the level of the group and not simply in terms of its individual members.

THE CONCEPT OF STRUCTURE

No understanding of groups is complete without an examination of the concept of *group structure*. Few human relationships are without structure. When we refer to the structure of a relationship or the structure of a group, we focus on the ways in which persons are involved in (a) ordered arrangements (b) that define and regulate their behavior and (c) that provide a patterned constancy and stability to their behavior together (Nadel, 1957).

Ordered Arrangements

In focusing on structure, we attempt to uncover the recurring patterns of relationship and interaction that exist without necessarily specifying who the persons are that participate in these ordered arrangements. There can be a total shift of personnel—old members leave and new members enter— yet the structural constraints on behavior remain the same. In music, for example, it is possible to speak about the structure of a symphony or the structure of a sonata without specifying the exact notes and melodies that are involved. Structure describes an arrangement of the parts (e.g., musical notes, group members, etc.) that is maintained regardless of what specific parts are involved.

For example, in an organization that is described as having a *tall* rather than a *flat* structure of authority and decision-making, persons on top make decisions that are handed down to those below (Porter & Lawler, 1964). The flat structure is more egalitarian; decision-making is shared among all persons rather than being handed down from the top. The terms "tall" and "flat" describe the power structure of the organization; regardless of what specific individuals are involved within it, they are constrained by the nature of the structure to behave in particular ways.

Constraints

The second part of this three-part definition of group structure calls attention to this defining and regulating (i.e., constraining) quality. If a composer were to write a sonata, for example, he or she would be constrained to use the structural arrangements that define the composition as a sonata regardless of the particular notes that were used. In a similar manner, the structure of a group defines and regulates the behavior of the persons involved in it. Persons high up in a tall organization are expected to exercise authority and hand down decisions just as those in a flat structure are expected to share more equally in decision-making.

To consider another example, the role structure of the society and its organizations (e.g., a hospital) defines a nurse's role and a doctor's role. To be sure, there may be variations in these definitions; certain aspects of the roles are more rigidly defined than other aspects. Nevertheless, a role description is a structural analysis. It informs us that regardless of which actual doctors and nurses are involved, they will be constrained by their roles to act in particular ways toward each other and toward their patients.

Knowing this structural feature of the relationship of the roles of nurse and doctor allows us to make some reasonable assessments of the behavior to expect even before we know which particular nurse and which particular doctor will actually be working together. Roles, however, compose only one of several structural features; we will shortly examine roles as well as the other important structural characteristics of groups. In all cases, however, the point remains: Structures are institutionally defined arrangements that regulate and constrain the behavior of whatever specific persons are involved working in them.

Stability

The third aspect of the definition of group structure informs us that structures provide a patterned constancy and stability to the behavior of the persons involved in the structure. Recall that structural properties of a group are defined independently of the particular persons who are members of the group; a change in membership thus need not produce a change in group structure. Constancy and stability are provided by the structural pattern rather than by any necessary constancy of personnel. A sonata is a sonata regardless of who has composed it, who performs it, and what notes are used in it. The constancy that permits us to recognize it as a sonata exists in and is carried by its musical structure.

It may be disconcerting to think in these terms. Nevertheless, it is important for the student of group process to understand that much that is constant and stable about group and individual behavior within groups is carried by the constancy of group structure rather than by a constancy of personnel. In very practical terms, this means that the personnel can be changed, many different personalities can be involved, and yet the group as such remains relatively constant and stable. A hospital is structurally similar and constant over time even when its personnel rotates out and even when the personalities of the specific individuals involved varies.

Structural Analysis

It should be apparent from our discussion of levels of analysis in (Chapter 3) that a structural analysis operates at the level of the group rather than the level of the individuals involved. What may not have been as apparent, however, is that our discussion of hospitalism in Chapter 1 illustrates what we mean when we discuss structural analysis. The constraints of a particular kind of hospital or unit structure, one in which staff members perform routine duties in a distant and formal way—technically proficient but humanly sterile—give rise to a behavioral syndrome called hospitalism. Our search for the bases of this syndrome must focus on the structural patterns within the organization that promote this behavior rather than on qualities within the personalities of either the patients or the staff. In many respects, even the most humane and concerned health professional who is placed within this type of organizational structure will in time come to take on many of the behavioral attributes of "hospitalism." Knowledge of group structure is thereby vital to the health professional who would both diagnose a group's problems and know something about the proper intervention strategy to employ.

Of course, there are limits to these constraints. A change in personnel, a unique coalescence of different personalities, can and does have consequences for the existing structure of a group or organization such as a hospital. New structures emerge as old structures are changed. In general, however, many of the constancies and the stabilities of behavior are carried by structures. Thus, even as the old structure gives way to the new—as persons bring new ways of interacting or as tasks demand different structures for their accomplishment—the new establishes its own ordered arrangements of the individuals who are working together.

Having considered the general concept of structure, we are in a position to apply it to some of the most typical structures one finds in groups.

We will first consider the role structures of groups and then examine communication, attraction, and power structures.

ROLE STRUCTURES

Of all the types of group structure, role structures are perhaps the most familiar and most easily understood (see Biddle & Thomas, 1966; Sarbin & Allen, 1968). This should come as no surprise. The concept of role is not used solely by sociologists or psychologists—it is a common term of analysis used by persons in their everyday dealings with one another. All societies, all groups, and all persons differentiate and classify populations into roles— that is, into positions that individuals take on and that carry with them certain expected behaviors and responsibilities (doctor, nurse, patient, teacher, director, mother, old man, woman, child, etc.).

Ascribed vs. Achieved Roles

Social scientists have found it useful to distinguish between two ways in which roles are classified (Linton, 1936). The first is termed *ascriptive*. *Ascribed roles* are based on certain characteristics that are intrinsic to the persons involved: e.g., male, female, young, old. The second involves *achievement*. *Achieved roles* are those that persons accomplish or achieve by virtue of their activities, things they do well, particular interests and abilities they have: e.g., doctor, nurse, president, etc. Not every instance of role behavior can be neatly classified as being either ascribed or achieved. The central emphasis, however, is clear. Ascribed roles are a function of some qualities that persons have that are generally beyond their control, such as their sex and their age. Achieved roles are a function of qualities over which they tend to have greater control, such as their occupation.

As with all structural characteristics, roles define and regulate the behavior of those who occupy them. Behavior is regulated by both our ascribed and our achieved roles. Sex and age, for example are ascribed characteristics that carry with them certain expectations for proper behavior; likewise, achieved roles define and constrain persons to certain proper behavior.

Fit Between Role and Self

Some roles fit certain people better than others. When there is a lack of fit between what the role demands and what the person feels capable of doing, we usually note symptoms of tension and discomfort both for the individual and for the particular role system (e.g., the group) in which the person is involved. For example, a supervisory position entails a role with expectations for the behavior of whoever occupies that position. If Adams is made supervisor, and acts in a withdrawn manner, hesitating to take the initiative to provide leadership and supervision, two consequences may fol-low. First, she may experience discomfort as she tries to behave in ways that fit the role's requirements but which do not fit her own personal ways of behaving. In time, she may grow into the role and become more the type of person it demands; or she may forever be at war with it. Second, the group may suffer when Adams does not enact her role properly. The role structure of a group usually consists of an interlocking network of several roles; when one or more does not function, the others in the network likewise have difficulty. The supervisor who does not take on the responsibilities proper to that role thereby leaves a gaping hole in the group's role structure.

Once again, a structural analysis (in this case, a role analysis) would be helpful both for understanding and intervening in a difficult group situa-tion. The supervisor in our example has a job that is ill-suited to her charac-ter. This creates problems for her and for her group. The source of the problem, however, is structural in that it involves the particular role con-straints that conflict with Adams's personality. Several options for change are now apparent. For example, Adams can delegate greater leadership responsibility to others; or she can try to work in a more egalitarian manner with the group. In this way, the group structure is changed from tall to flat and thereby the supervisory role is transformed from one requiring greater dominance to one requiring a more democratic arrangement. Thus we see that a recognition of the structural basis of a problem can help in bringing about a structural solution.

Conflict Between Different Roles

All of us occupy more than one role; we may be mother or father and doctor; we may be teacher by day and student by night. We can usually avoid the difficulties involved in having to enact both roles simultaneously by segregating them in time or in place. For example, we can be parent at home and nurse at work; we do our parenting at one time and fulfill our obliga-tions as nurse at another time. There are moments, however, when a conflict develops between the several roles we occupy. This conflict may occur, for example, when the same job is defined differently for us by the different persons with whom we interact; that is, our role means one thing to one person and something different to another. We are placed in a conflict, then, between these differing conceptions of our role. In a sense, it is a conflict between two sets of roles.

The classic example of this conflict occurs for people who occupy middle-level positions within an organization (Stouffer et al., 1949a, b). Those who are superior to them in the organization's hierarchy define their role in one way, usually seeing them as representative of the administrative hierarchy; those who are below them in the organization define their role in a very different way, usually seeing them as a friend, one of their own group. There is little chance for people caught in the middle to segregate their roles by time or place; they are both, at the same time and in the same place.

One version of this conflict between two roles is highlighted by the following example:

> A nursing supervisor enrolled for a course in interviewing and counseling techniques, hoping to learn how to better deal with what she felt to be a difficult situation. As supervisor, she was expected to be a rather stern, authoritative person, making certain that the young nurses under her supervision got their work done properly. Yet she was also expected to provide these younger and less experienced nurses with a warm and supportive figure to whom they could turn in their own moments of need and personal crisis. The nursing supervisor complained that she just didn't know how to take on both of these conflicting roles at the same time. How could she be both stern/authoritative and warm/supportive?

As was noted earlier, roles are so interlocked that a problem for the role occupant becomes a problem for everyone tied into that same role relationship. In the case of the nursing supervisor, not only did she face a problem, but so too did all the nurses she was supervising. Who was she from their perspective? Let us suppose that they had problems and wanted to seek some support from her. When they approached her, how could they know which role she was enacting? Was she the stern figure who would reject their claims for support as she tried to get them to do their work more efficiently? Or was she the warm figure to whom they could turn for a shoulder to cry on and support for their confusion? Her problem, in other words, was their problem as well.

It is reasonable to refer to the kinds of conflict expressed in the previous example as *structural*. Any person who occupies roles of the sort described would experience conflict. The conflict is built into the structure of the group or organization; in this regard, therefore, it is not like the conflict between self and role. The latter entails conflict for only certain kinds of persons. To recognize something as involving a structural conflict rather than a more personal one can often alleviate some of the strains that people feel. Rather than always putting the blame on themselves, they can see the structural context within which the conflict is generated. To be sure, the pain and anguish will not thereby be magically dissipated, but seeing its origin in structural terms can help considerably.

Understanding the nature of conflict in structural rather than in personal terms can also provide a clue as to its resolution. A structural conflict will not fade simply with psychotherapy or a happy attitude toward one's work; such conflicts require a solution that attacks the proper level of the problem: that is, a structural solution is required. Organizational changes are required to alleviate the personal problems that derive from these kinds of structural arrangements. On the other hand, where the organization remains resistant to change or where the efforts involved in seeking to affect such change seem beyond one's abilities, the best tactic may be to bite the bullet and bear the structural conflict or get out. Because few conflicts are purely personal or purely structural, a compromise between changing one's own outlook somewhat and seeking to somewhat modify the organizational structure may work best in the long run.

Group Roles

Analysts of group process have noted role structures in all groups, including both formal groups that emphasize task functions and informal groups that emphasize more social functions. Role structures in groups often overlap with the prevailing communication and power structures. For example, the differentiation between group leader and members describes a feature of both the group's role structure and its power structure. Similarly, an analysis of members into roles based on their predominant mode of communicating and interacting proves informative about both the role structure and the communication structure of the group. Research reported by Bales (1958) has suggested two major roles within all groups based on the types of communication that describe the particular role. He refers to these as *task roles* and socioemotional or *maintenance roles*.

Task and Social Specialists

Bales's analysis argues that all groups must develop role structures in order to deal with two kinds of problems: the external problem of successfully coping with the task they have undertaken; and the internal problem of successfully dealing with inter-member relations. Specialty roles tend to emerge within groups to handle each type of problem. A *task specialist* has to do with a role or set of roles that emphasize getting the job done, working in ways that are more efficient for dealing with the group's tasks. A *social specialist* involves a role or set of roles that emphasize keeping the group working together in relative harmony, dealing with conflicts with the group, and generally helping with issues of group maintenance.

Based on their own and others' observations of many groups, Benne and Sheats (1948) expanded somewhat on Bales's analysis. They not only described further types of roles within the task and the group maintenance areas, but in addition they introduced a third set of roles involving what they termed *individual functions*. This third category includes roles that serve individual members' own personal needs rather than those of the group as a whole. Table 4-1 summarizes several examples of their role analysis.

As with Bales's analysis, the roles proposed by Benne and Sheats suggest an aspect of group structure in which any number of group members may participate. Dr. Winslow, for example, may take on the individualistic role of dominator in one session and take on the task role of initiator in another. Nurse Coopersmith might serve the task function of coordinator in one session or one part of a group meeting and take on the maintenance role of harmonizer in another part of that same meeting or in another session. These describe patterned ways of behaving within groups and not necessarily particular people. Naturally, a given individual may characteristically adopt one kind of role or another. Thus, Nurse Coopersmith may typically take on a mixture of task and maintenance functions, while Dr. Winslow typically functions within the individualistic area.

Table 4-1. Member Roles Within Groups

Roles Involving Task Functions

Initiator: involves proposing new ideas, new directions, new tasks, new methods.

Elaborator: involves expanding on existing suggestions, developing further meanings to the group's plans.

Evaluator: involves critically evaluating ideas, proposals, and plans, examining the practicality of proposals, the effectiveness of procedures.

Coordinator: involves helping to pull ideas and themes together, to clarify suggestions that have been made, to help various subgroups work more effectively together toward their common goals.

Roles Involving Group Maintenance Functions

Encourager: involves offering praise and agreement with other members; involves communicating acceptance of others and their ideas and an openness to differences within the group.

Harmonizer: involves mediating conflicts and disagreements that crop up, trying to relieve or reduce tension within the group.

Compromiser: involves seeking a position between contending sides, seeking a compromise that all parties can accept.

Roles Involving Primarily Personal, Individualistic Functions

Aggressor: involves acting negatively, with hostility toward other members, denigrating others' contributions, attacking the group and its members.

Recognition-Seeker: involves efforts to call attention to one's own activities, to boast, to redirect things toward oneself.

Help-seeker or confessor: involves using the group as a vehicle either to gain sympathy or to accomplish personal insights and personal satisfactions without consideration for others or the group as a whole.

Dominator: involves asserting authority and seeking to manipulate others so as to be in control of everything that happens.

What is important to understand about Bales's analysis and that of Benne and Sheats is that role structures emerge within a group in order to serve certain basic functions that are necessary for the group's success. Some functions are concerned with getting the external task completed, while other functions are concerned with maintaining the group while it works together. Both sets of functions must be served for the group to be effective. Individualistic roles do not serve these necessary group functions, but rather serve member's personal needs often at the expense of the group.

When Bales speaks of a role specialist such as a task specialist, he is refer-ring to a set of communicative behaviors that attend to task functions. These behaviors involve some of the specific activities that Benne and Sheats list under their category: e.g., initiating, elaborating, evaluating, coordinating. While these two sets of functions, task and maintenance, must be served and roles must emerge to deal with them, the particular individuals who come forward to serve them can vary. As with all aspects of group structure, the specific personnel may change within a group, but these two functions and the roles that serve them remain.

The Gatekeeper

Lewin's analysis (1958) of the use of group processes in behavior main-tenance and change (recall Chapter 1) introduces us to another role within groups: that of *gatekeeper*. It was Lewin's suggestion that a key role within any group is the one that provides an entry point from the outside into the group. In the examples he studied, involving changing the eating habits of families, he suggested that the wife was the gatekeeper to the family's dinner table. That is, she was in the key position to determine what food was actually served. Thus, to affect a change in the gatekeeper would be to affect a change in the entire family's eating habits.

The student of group process, especially in the health professions, must be sensitive to this type of group role. To find the gatekeeper of a group is to find the key role that permits the outsider (e.g., the health professional) entry into the group. As in Lewin's own example, in many families, the health-care issues are focused around the wife and mother as the gatekeeper. It is she, therefore, who occupies the critical position within the family when it comes to making health-related decisions. This may not be true in all fami-lies; but identifying the gatekeeper is critical for anyone who needs to work with that group.

In many instances, group leaders may need to know who is the gatekeeper to an informal clique or subgroup within their own larger group in order to have effective access to all members of the group. For example, a health professional team may consist of eight persons, three of whom could be said to form a subgroup of close friends within the larger group of eight. To work most effectively with the entire group, the team's leader would benefit from knowing who was the gatekeeper to that three-person subgroup. To reach that gatekeeper and influence his or her behavior would be the most effec-tive way to reach all members of the subgroup. Indeed, as we can recall from Lewin's analysis in Chapter 1, trying to influence a member of that subgroup without due consideration for the dynamics of the subgroup, especially its organization around the gatekeeper, might prove to be a wasted effort.

As in the other cases we have been considering, a structural role analysis proves to be an essential first step in planning and carrying out intervention into a group. Much time and effort are wasted by a health professional, for example, who makes contact with a family through one of the less influential members rather than the gatekeeper. It may be possible to convince that person of the need for a change in the family's health practices, but this may not be effective in producing a change for the entire family. Here the failure lies primarily in not first determining the role structure of the family so that time and effort can be invested in the most fruitful direction.

Much the same type of approach is necessary within organizations as well. A health professional who wishes to introduce a change procedure on a particular unit may get the agreement of some staff, but fail to get the change accepted by the entire unit. This may be due to the failure to examine the structure of the unit first, in order to determine who the gatekeeper for that unit is.

COMMUNICATION STRUCTURES

Communication between persons tends to be structured in various ways. Even within a conversation, we can readily note aspects of the communication structure that is involved.

> Head Nurse Fields, with some fifteen years of experience behind her, addresses all the other nurses on her unit by their first name, except when in the presence of patients; then, she addresses them by their last name—e.g., Riley. She prefers to be addressed always by her title and last name: Mrs. Fields. When she speaks with the doctors, however, she uses their title and last name under all circumstances; she would never think of calling a doctor by his or her first name, even in private, in spite of the difference in their ages and years of experience.

The way we address others, using their first name, their last name, or their title and last name—where Dr., Mrs., Mr. and Ms. are examples of title—is an aspect of the structure of communication within a conversation that we all employ (Ervin-Tripp, 1969). In the example, we note several informative aspects of this structure. For example, we see that the head nurse addresses the other nurses on her unit by their first names (when not in the patients' presence), but expects to be referred to by her own title and last name under all circumstances. The form of address exchanged by two or more persons reveals something about the status relationships that exist between them. Research (Brown & Ford, 1961; Brown & Gilman, 1960) has shown that status equals exchange first names or exchange last names without titles (e.g., Hi, Riley; Hi, Fields), whereas status unequals differ in the structure of their communications: those in status-superior positions expect to be addressed with title and last name while addressing status inferiors by their first name.

Another structural feature revealed in the example involves the head nurse's use of title and last name when addressing the doctors. Even though their experience may be far less than hers, they represent status superiority within the hospital situation. This is reflected in the structure of communication used to address them. Finally, the head nurse does not use first names when addressing the other nurses on her unit if patients are present. This also reflects an aspect of the communication structure involved. Patients fall outside the hospital's status system, but are dealt with in more formal, impersonal ways; thus she feels that it is not appropriate for them to hear the less formal, more personal use of first names.

Networks

Communication structures within groups involve the patterns of communication that take place within the group. The observer of communication will note that not everyone speaks to everyone else, nor, as the illustrative case indicates, not everyone uses the same forms (e.g., of address) when communicating to others. There are patterned flows to the communication that takes place; we can literally see channels that are open to communication and channels that are closed.

The experimental laboratory permits us to intentionally create these various channels of communication in order to study their effects (Bavelas, 1950; Leavitt, 1958). An example of three such channels in a five-person group is presented in Figure 4-1.

Figure 4-1. Illustrates three arrangements of communication that are possible within this five-person group. The circle describes a communication structure in which messages are readily communicated around to everyone. In the chain, messages eventually get around to everyone but there are several intervening steps to be crossed. In the wheel, messages get around but only by passing through the most central position, in this example, the head nurse.

Centrality

This is one of the key structural features of communication networks such as those illustrated. In the wheel, the most highly central position is the head nurse. In the chain, the doctor and the nursing assistant both occupy the least central positions, being the farthest removed from ready communication with other members of the group. In the circle, all persons are equally central, being the same distance from everyone else.

Research with *simple* laboratory tasks (Leavitt, 1958) has shown that the wheel is the most efficient arrangement for simple problem-solving; the chain is next and the circle is the least efficient. However, as the complexity of the task increases, especially as it requires decision-making and the evaluation of alternatives, then the circle proves to be the most efficient structure (Smith, 1951). In fact, with a complex group task, the wheel may be the least efficient, producing the worst decisions if the central person is not very capable or if the peripheral members with good ideas never get a chance to have them evaluated by others in their group. Research (Leavitt, 1958) has also shown that with simple tasks, group morale and a sense of satisfaction is highest in the circle, where all are equally involved, and least high in the wheel, where one member's centrality dominates and leaves the others out of the picture.

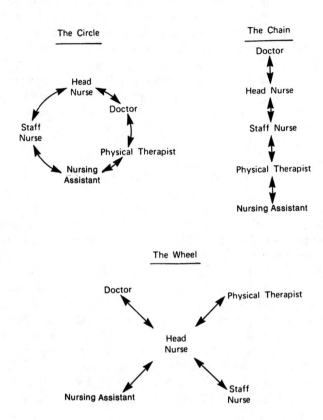

Figure 4-1.   Three sample communication structures within groups.

While most "real" groups do not appear to be as rigidly structured as those represented in Figure 4-1, there are sufficient parallels to warrant our careful consideration. Persons occupying different positions within a group may indeed never communicate directly with one another; they may always communicate through an intermediary. Or the group's leader may arrange things so that only he or she gains access to all the information needed for decision-making, keeping the others more or less in the dark as in the wheel-type structure. Under such circumstances, the competence of this most central person can significantly affect the group's efficiency. For example, a less competent leader can harm the group more when he or she occupies the most central position and thereby receives and evaluates all information and then hands down decisions (the work of Hyrcenko & Minton, 1974, provides a relevant example). In addition, such a highly centralized arrangement does not give others the opportunity to provide checks and balances on their own or on others' suggestions. The burden is put entirely on the leader's shoulders. We return to this theme in the chapter on leadership (Chapter 12).

Although the structures in Figure 4-1 may appear to be rather rigid, they are often reflected in actual groups, especially within organizations such as hospitals and especially as such groups bring together persons of differing social standing. Even less formal groups, including primary groups (e.g., families and informal work teams) have a discernible communication structure. Recall that a structure exists whenever we are able to note a pattern of communication that has some stability and continuity even when the persons are exchanged.

ATTRACTION STRUCTURES

Let us suppose that members of a group are asked to name several people in their group that they most like or feel most friendly toward. Let us further suppose that these answers are tallied and the results represented in a diagram. Figure 4-2 provides one possible arrangement of "liking" choices for a group. The circles with initials represent members of the group. The arrows represent directions of choosing: e.g., KL→ML means that KL lists ML as one of his or her most liked persons.

Figure 4-2 indicates several interesting structural features based on "liking" or attraction. First we note that one person, SN, appears to be what Moreno (1951; 1953) has called a *sociometric star*. This is a person who occupies a central position in terms of being chosen as most liked by most of the others in the group. An unchosen person, or *sociometric isolate*, in this diagram is represented by MR. Though MR chooses one other, he or she is unchosen by anyone else in the group.

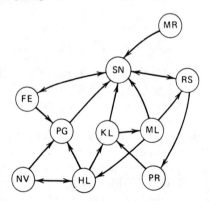

Figure 4-2. The attraction structure of a group.

We can notice another feature of this group's attraction structure. Several choices are *mutual*, suggesting a pairing of members into subgroups: e.g.,

SN and FE; SN and RS; NV and HL. We also notice, however, that many choices are not reciprocated: e.g., PG is chosen by HL but does not reciprocate the choice; KL is chosen by PR but does not reciprocate. Finally, we can note the existence of *pathways* through the liking structure; these pathways link persons together through liked intermediaries: e.g., PR chooses KL who chooses SN who chooses RS who chooses PR. We have other pathways that unlike this circular one, do not return to their point of origin: e.g., HL chooses KL, who chooses SN.

Knowing the attraction structure of a group can provide us with some important information about that group: the morale and level of satisfaction of certain individuals; the alienation of other individuals; the probable pattern and flow of communication within the group; the power and influence structure of the group. Sociometric stars tend to be more satisfied and isolates more alienated. Communication tends to follow the attraction structure: persons linked by liking relationship tend to communicate more with one another. Furthermore, information that enters the group from the outside is likely to flow along the liking pathways. For example, getting some information to NV can result in its flow to HL and PG. From those two, the information branches throughout much of the group. Finally, there tends to be a relation between liking and influence; persons who are well-liked tend to be more influential within the group than isolates. Thus, knowing the attraction structure of the group can prove informative about its influence structure as well.

Another component of the attraction structure that is relevant involves the degree of reciprocation or nonreciprocation that characterizes an entire group. Where many group members choose others but are not chosen by them in return, we can expect problems of group morale, cohesiveness, and effectiveness in coordinated work. In such a group, people may not perceive one another very clearly; they may send out liking but fail to note that it is not reciprocated; they may feel they have a good relationship with others in their group only to realize one day that this is a faulty perception. This can be damaging to individual self-esteem as well as to group morale.

POWER STRUCTURES

Most groups, including both formal and informal, both primary and secondary, can be characterized by their structures of power, influence, and authority. Families, for example, although defined as primary groups, have their own characteristic power structures. A traditional family is defined in terms of a rather distinct power hierarchy, with the father heading the household and the wife and children "lower" in power. The less traditional, more contemporary family is also characterized by its power structure; in this case, the structure reveals greater equality between husband and wife than in the traditional family. In addition, in many household matters, this modern family form may give children near equality in decision-making influence with the parents.

Other informal groups also have a structure of power, although it may be one that shifts about more than in traditional family groups or in more formally structured groups. Think of some informal groups in which you are a member. Whose decisions seem to carry the most weight when you are all deciding about something to do together? Who is listened to most? Which members elicit the most attentiveness from the others when they speak? Which members elicit the least attention? These are all questions whose answers can help reveal the structure of power and influence within even informal groups.

Within more formal groups, the structuring of power and influence tends to be relatively stable and relatively well-known by all the participants. An investigation reported by Zander, Cohen, and Stotland in 1957, for example, studied the power structure among mental health teams composed of psychiatrists, psychologists, and psychiatric social workers. Their data indicate the not-too-surprising fact that all groups recognize a pecking order with the psychiatrists on top, the psychologists next, and the social workers third. And there was substantial agreement within each group as to this relative ranking in terms of power and influence.

Needless to say, any organization composed of highly trained specialists, each carrying out specific duties involved with patient diagnosis and care, has a relatively stable power structure that varies by profession (e.g., doctors have more authority than R.N.s), by position within profession (supervisor has more authority than staff); and even by such variables as sex within profession (e.g., males tend to be higher in power and authority than females even within the same profession, even though this too is changing); and prestige outside the organization (e.g., doctors with national reputations tend to gain greater power within the organization than other doctors).

Lest the incorrect picture emerge, we should note that a power structure for a group need not indicate one-way influence. That is, once we have mapped out the hierarchy of power and influence of a group, this mapping does not mean that the position on top has license to do whatever he or she pleases, giving influence and exercising authority but receiving little in return. As we will note in more detail in Chapters 10 and 12, the exercise of power is a two-way street; the successful use of power requires an evaluation of factors that resist its acceptance as well. Thus, knowing the power structure of a group does not necessarily inform us about how successful that group is; nor are we informed about how successful the person with the most power is in getting the things accomplished that he or she wishes. But knowing the structure of power and authority of a group does reveal a great deal that we must know if we are to work effectively with the group. Since power and authority overlap so extensively with issues of leadership, we will leave a further discussion of these issues to Chapter 12.

SUMMARY AND CONCLUSIONS

The chapter has dealt with the structural aspects of groups. Structure refers to ordered arrangements that constrain behavior and that provide it with a constancy and stability. Structure is a property of groups and relationships that exists relatively independently of the particular individuals who are involved. Thus, for example, we noted that a group may have a tall (i.e., hierarchical) or a flat (i.e., egalitarian) leadership and power structure that exists as a property of the group separate from the personalities of particular members. We examined several important structural features of groups, including role structures, communication structures, attraction structures, and power structures.

5

Group Norms

*A*ll groups—formal and informal, primary and secondary—have sets of standards for the behavior, attitudes, and even the perceptions of their members. These standards are called the *norms* of the group: shared expectations for what is appropriate and inappropriate behavior, what members should and shouldn't do. All groups not only have norms—they also have mechanisms whereby conformity to these norms is accomplished, ways in which group pressures are brought to bear on members who stray too far from the group's norms.

The *content* of the norms tends to vary from group to group, as does the degree to which the norms are *explicit* or *implicit*. Groups also vary in the form that normative pressures take, in the intensity of these pressures, and in the targets of these normative pressures: i.e., who in the group is permitted more or less leeway in following the norms.

EXTENSITY

There are some groups in which the content of the norms cover all aspects of the members' lives. Membership in some religious groups, for example, carries along with it expectations for nearly all behaviors and attitudes that members should have. The content of such norms, thus, is extensive, directing members' manner of dress, their private behavior, their public attitudes and conduct, and so forth. On the other hand, occupational groups, especially in complex societies, tend to emphasize normative content that centers more on job-related issues. Members' private lives are usually not under the direction of occupational group norms; rather, such behavior tends to be encompassed by the norms of people's informal, family, and friendship groups.

Medical and health specialties often formulate group norms for members that extend widely, encompassing the members' private lives. These norms often involve ethical issues, outlining behaviors that health professionals should and should not engage in within their professional practice as well as their private lives. Medical and other health professionals are also typically under wide-ranging normative pressure to be willing to sacrifice much of their own personal and private life (especially time) to their profession. Teachers, for example, may be expected to put in a work week of generally defined and limited hours; it is usually considered appropriate for them to resist efforts to cut into their personal time. Health professionals, however, typically have less personal time and greater expectations to be on call and available; they can properly make some efforts to protect their private moments, but in general, normative expectations allow them less free time than other occupational groups.

Within the typical work group or health professional team, the content of group norms typically focuses on work-related issues: e.g., the appropriate tasks for the members; the ways members interact with one another both on and off the job; the way patients are dealt with; the kinds of clothing that should and shouldn't be worn; the perspectives on treatment; the extent of openness and trust among members; the formality or informality of relationships within the group; the type of leadership style legitimate for the group; and so forth.

EXPLICITNESS

In noting that norms may be explicit or implicit, we wish to call attention to the fact that some groups have stated an explicit set of guidelines for proper member behavior; at times, these are presented to new members who are to learn them as part of their induction into the group. Other groups, though having many norms and standards for members' behavior, are much less explicit about these. These norms appear as an implicit, shared understanding that members have about what is and what is not appropriate behavior. Even groups with a set of very explicit norms also tend to have many implicit understandings. Thus a new member may learn the explicit set of rules rather readily, but may require much additional time before he or she can grasp these implicit understandings. A new nurse, for example, may violate the implicit norms of her team by asking too many questions; though this is never stated as an explicit group norm, in time she learns that question-asking is a behavior that this team regulates and feels should be kept to a minimum.

One way to determine the norms of a group is to ask the members (including oneself as a member), "What is considered appropriate and what is considered inappropriate behavior for members of this group?" For example, if a member is late for a meeting (or in a family, if someone arrives late to dinner), would that be considered appropriate or inappropriate? Are there rules or opinions about being on time in this group? In conducting even so simple an exercise, it may be surprising to discover the number of norms that exist within any one group, the content that is covered by these norms, and the degree to which they are explicit.

CONFORMITY

Conformity to norms, while expected in all groups, is handled differently in different groups. Even within the same group, normative pressures (i.e., group pressures to conform to the norm) are handled differently for different members. Groups have several ways to achieve conformity to norms. For the most part, other than using threatened or actual physical restraint or punishment—an approach that characterizes some families, some classrooms, some military and athletic groups, and some institutionalized groups—the more usual approaches involve verbal influence, including praising or reproaching members, and rejection, even to the point of actual ostracism from the group.

The potency of most norms, however, is their quality of being understood without members always having to test them out and receive punishment. Conformity to group norms becomes rewarding in itself to the group's members. They feel good about behaving in ways that are considered appropriate by their group and feel guilt or shame when behaving inappropriately. Members are rewarded by the acceptance of their fellow members when they follow norms; often, higher prestige and status within the group hinges on members' behaving in ways that live up to the group's standards.

For example, on a particular team, there is an unspoken but shared norm regarding innovation in developing care plans for patients. A student who is innovative in giving and in recommending care is praised by other team members; his or her status rises within the group and the level of acceptance by others is increased. Deviancy does not earn much esteem from fellow members. Much conformity to group norms occurs without actual punishment ever having to be undertaken.

IDIOSYNCRASY CREDIT

Not all members are subjected to the same kinds of normative pressure or sanction for having violated the norms. Although the research on this point is not completely firm in its conclusions, there are indications that persons of higher status within a group can deviate from norms with relative impunity as compared with members of lesser status. Coming in late for dinner, for example, may bring harsh punishment for a child but little repercussion for the father. Or the chairperson who has called the group together may arrive late with little punishment whereas anyone arriving after that person may be considered late and treated accordingly. In most medical settings, a physician can arrive late to a scheduled meeting with relative impunity; on the other hand, a student or a staff nurse arriving late meets with disapproval or even direct punishment.

Hollander (1958; 1961) introduced the concept of *idiosyncrasy credit* to refer to one aspect of this issue. He suggested that members who dutifully follow their group's norms not only earn higher prestige within the group as examples of what a "good" member is but also build up a credit against future deviance: These are termed idiosyncrasy credits. In this view, a person with a high "credit rating" can behave idiosyncratically in violation of group norms with relative impunity. When the credit runs out, however, conformity to group standards is again expected. Members who are new to a group or who have never built up much credit are those most likely to be sanctioned for any departures from appropriate behavior.

If a person were to adopt this concept as a self-conscious policy for behavior, then he or she would spend some initial time in a new group building up credits by conforming fully to group norms. These early credits could then be spent later. The staff nurse who always shows up at meetings on time and in other ways earns a reputation as a good group member may gain greater leeway than the person who has never built up credits in the first place.

VISIBILITY AND PRESSURE

Groups and roles within groups often vary in the degree to which behaviors are open to observation and evaluation by other members or outsiders. This describes the *visibility* of the group or role. A role with high visibility is one in which the person's performance is open to the scrutiny and evaluation of others. With low visibility, one cannot be evaluated as readily by others, and thus conformity to group norms is less easily determined. Visibility is related to group norms and normative pressures; less visibility permits greater deviation from normative expectations. Basically, those behaviors that are more open to the surveillance and evaluation of others permit less leeway for deviation from group norms when compared with behaviors that are low in their visibility. Arriving late for a meeting is a behavior of high visibility and thus is readily open to sanctions. The job attitude a person has, however, tends to be of lesser visibility. Even though group norms may demand that members all share a high level of enthusiasm for their work, any member can feel little enthusiasm without being the recipient of group sanctions for this "invisible" deviant attitude. Of course, if the attitude leaks into a public display or obvious discontent and low motivation, then sanctions are likely.

THE FUNCTION OF NORMS AND
NORMATIVE PRESSURES

Norms do not simply arise within groups nor do pressures to conform to these norms simply evolve for the sake of making life more troublesome for members who would be free spirits. Analysts of group process have suggested several important functions served by norms and normative pressures.

Task Functions

On the one hand, a hypothetical, purely fictional group that sought to function without any normative regulation of members' behavior would give meaning to the idea of chaos. One critical function that norms serve is to permit groups to function in relatively coordinated ways in the accomplishment of their tasks and goals. We would expect, therefore, that the most explicit statement of norms and the greatest pressure for conformity to such norms would converge around the task functions of goal attainment, at least in groups for which task achievement is the critical purpose for existence. Groups that are organized around more social functions, on the other hand, may play down goal achievement and emphasize norms that deal with members' interpersonal styles, openness, friendliness compatibility, and so forth.

Maintenance Functions

A second function that norms and normative pressures serve falls more directly in the group maintenance area. Not all groups will emphasize maintenance issues, but the problem of group maintenance exists whenever two or more persons convene for whatever purpose. Thus we would expect to find norms developing around maintenance issues such as attendance at group meetings, standards about how disagreements are to be expressed and resolved, behaviors involving conflict and its resolution, standards involving members' personal relations, and so forth.

Social Reality Functions

A critical third function that group norms and normative pressures serve involves what have been called *social reality functions* (Festinger, 1954; Schachter, 1951). Most of the issues with which each of us deal in our daily lives at work and elsewhere confront us with matters that involve the interpretation of facts. In measuring blood pressure, for example, the factual matter involves the reading on the gauge. This is something that we can determine relatively independently of others and with little interpretation required. However, the decision about what that reading means and what the next step in the diagnostic procedure should be, begins to converge on matters of interpretation. We choose the word "interpretation" rather than "opinion" in order to emphasize that the arena of social reality is not simply one of opinion about this or that matter; rather, social reality pertains to the interpretation that persons make of even hard facts and hard data. Thus, interpretation extends throughout all facets of our living and practice.

In matters of interpretation, judgments must be made regarding the status of reality. The gauge reads 120/80, but what does this mean? The reality in such interpretative matters is embedded in social contexts; thus it is referred to as a social reality as distinct from the sheer physical reality of the reading on the gauge. To say that reality is social is to note that the evaluation of its truth or falsity is social; that is, it depends on agreements of interpretation rendered by others with whom we associate, including others who publish in scholarly journals and whose analyses become accepted as facts.

Perceptual Facts

To say that reality is social is to emphasize the group processes that are involved in constituting and creating what we take to be real, true, and valid (Berger & Luckman, 1966). Much laboratory research in social psychology has been concerned with examining how group norms develop in the service of providing persons with a sense of a shared social reality, even in matters that ostensibly appear not to require an extensive interpretation. The early work of Asch, (1952) for example, showed how persons would actually change their own perception or verbal reports about the length of a line presented to them after they heard the estimate provided by other members of their group. Thus members were influenced to see or to report their own judgment of the line's length so as not to depart too much from the estimates given by others in their group. Deutsch and Gerard (1955) later demonstrated that the more the individuals felt themselves to be members of a group—that is, the more interdependent they were—the more extensive was the effect of the group's normative judgments on the individual's own estimates.

Frame of Reference

In more ambiguous settings, others (Sherif, 1935) have demonstrated how groups provide a judgmental frame of reference or norm within which members come to evaluate the status of reality. In Sherif's work, the reality involved the distance a point of light apparently moved in a darkened room. Over a period of some time together, groups developed a standard for judging this distance; once a standard emerged, it provided the framework within which members came to perceive the light's movement. For example, in one group the consensus developed that the light was moving somewhere in the range of 2 to 5 inches. This served as a framework within which individuals came to make their own assessments of its movement. Thus, a member would report his or her judgment somewhere within that 2- to 5-inch standard; to report something smaller or greater than that range would be to deviate from the group's standard or norm of judgment regarding the light's movement. In similar fashion, group norms provide the frame of reference within which we make our own judgments about social reality.

Resistance

In the many critical matters of social reality, the touchstone by which we gauge our own interpretations about what is and what is not correct, true, or real is given by the groups to which we belong or whose views we have come to accept as offering us a valid perspective (Newcomb, 1958; 1961; Newcomb et al., 1967). Many group norms thereby offer the individual social definitions and interpretations of reality. Normative pressures involve ways of dealing with potentially threatening challenges to these shared definitions of reality. Members who stray too far from the group's norms cast doubt on the validity of the interpretations that are used to understand social reality. It is difficult to be open and hospitable to such challenges. Not surprisingly, some of the strongest normative pressures are brought to bear whenever the deviation pertains to this social reality function.

For example, the resistance of a team of health professionals to a new procedure or technique often involves the implication that adherents to the old way are thereby incorrect or misguided in their views regarding diagnosis or patient care. New discoveries that open old practices to doubt are often met with resistance and even rejection.

Resistance to innovation can occur when a new practice involves something as simple and noncontroversial as the use of a team approach in the treatment of selected surgical patients. For instance, Mrs. Watts will require colostomy surgery. Should a rehabilitation team of health professionals consisting of a physician, a nurse-specialist, a nutritionist, a physical therapist, a psychologist, and a social worker be developed to work with Mrs. Watts and her family throughout the surgical procedure and afterward? In this case, resistance may develop around the very idea of a team approach.

Some medical specialists may doubt that a team approach is appropriate in this case. In their view, she will undergo surgery and will only require a few follow-up visits. The idea of a team of health professionals to develop and carry out a treatment plan for her and her family is the kind of innovation that may meet resistance. As we probe the basis of this resistance, we realize that it implies something about the validity of the old practice: that is, the implication is that a team approach is necessary because the old way is not satisfactory. And this implication is a clear threat to those with vested interests in the old ways of practice; thus, much of their resistance is based on the threats to their concepts of what medical reality in the treatment of cancer is all about.

But it need not be a new procedure or a new discovery. A new group member may bring with her the practices of her former groups and meet great resistance from the new group: "We don't do things that way around here."

Nurse Arlington has attended several human sexuality workshops and is concerned with the sexuality issues that are involved in nursing and medical practice. In an effort to determine more about these issues, she begins to make some informal inquiries of her co-workers on her new job at City Hospital. The group on her former unit and her sexuality training groups all had norms in which the discussion of sexuality was a rather routine matter; people were encouraged to talk openly and nondefensively about sexual feelings, impulses, ideas, practices, myths, and so forth as they were relevant to patient care. Nurse Arlington believes nothing is unusual, therefore, about making the same kind of inquiries on her new job. She is quite mistaken. Although no one directly approaches her and says, "Those questions are not appropriate around here" (another norm

of this new group involves never confronting others directly with disagreements)
she is made to realize in any number of indirect ways that her questions are
a violation of her new group's standards.

As we try to understand the basis for the group's resistance to Nurse Arlington's questioning, we discover the social reality function that underlies their
norms against uncovering issues of sexuality.

The group as a whole does not resist Nurse Arlington's questioning
because it pertains to sexual issues, although some individual members may
do so. More significantly, the resistance occurs because the content falls outside the group's definition of what is relevant (i.e., real, true, valid, correct)
for medical and nursing practice. The group has shared definitions of nursing and medical practice that excludes issues of sexuality in much the same
way that astrological or political issues are excluded from their definitions
of social reality relevant to health care.

Nurse Arlington's questioning about sexuality casts doubt upon the
groups' exclusion of what they may suspect to be an important concern to
their practice but one which thus far they have refused to confront. Their
resistance reflects the problems that including her ideas into their own analysis would entail: e.g., everyone would have to become familiar with human
sexuality and its relation to their practice as health professionals; they might
even have to rethink their own practices and dramatically revise some of
their procedures.

The Social Basis of Reality

Of all the functions that norms and normative pressures serve, the social
reality function is perhaps one of the most complex and least understood
by most practitioners. Basically, we must realize that much of what we know
and accept to be true and valid is socially determined. We accept as matters
of fact many matters of social interpretation. We search for those groups
that provide confirmation for our ways of interpreting and knowing reality;
we pressure those whose alternative interpretations challenge our own; we
ask them to leave or to be quiet so that we need not open up our own views
of reality to excessive doubt. All groups have evolved their own normative
definitions and interpretations of reality; and all groups bring pressures to
bear on members to remain within the fold of their views.

Not too surprisingly, people leave groups when competing perspectives
on social reality force them to meet the challenge by adopting another group's
analysis. Not surprisingly, people join groups whose points of view mesh relatively closely with their own. And not surprisingly, we all participate in bringing normative pressures to bear on those who seem to violate our collective
sense of the right and proper reality. In that interpretative issues pervade
all of our practice—that is, no matter how factual the base of our practice,
the context of meaning within which to interpret those facts is socially
rooted—the social reality function of group norms and normative
pressures likewise pervades much of what we do.

INTENSITY OF NORMATIVE PRESSURES

Research (Schachter, 1951) has suggested two important factors that affect the intensity of the pressures for members to adopt and follow group norms: *relevance* and *cohesiveness*.

Relevance

Relevance refers to the idea that group norms can vary in their importance to a group's task functions, its maintenance functions, or its social reality functions. The greater the relevance of the norm to any of these functions, the greater will be the pressure on members to follow that norm. For example, if the task of a group is to meet and plan a curriculum for in-service training, group norms that involve the way members should dress at the meetings would appear less relevant to that task and thus less likely to involve normative pressures than matters more central to the task at hand: e.g., how competing philosophies of nursing will be expressed and resolved by the group. We are all aware, however, of seemingly irrelevant matters that can become of great concern to a group. Issues of social reality and group maintenance have a way of encompassing many content areas. The way a member dresses for a curriculum committee meeting, for example, may be "read" by the group leader as a sign of commitment to the group or as rejection of the group and its goals. Thus, even clothing might be considered highly relevant. In general, however, once we have determined areas and functions that are of high and low relevance to a particular group, then we can know what behaviors are most and least likely to receive normative pressures. And much of this determination is based on the purposes and goals of the group.

Cohesiveness

We previously encountered the concept of cohesiveness in Chapter 3 we saw that it refers to the members' attraction to their group. This attraction can be based on several things (Cartwright & Zander, 1968):

—Attraction to the *members* of the group

—Attraction to the *task* of the group

—Attraction to the *goals and ideals* of the group

Whatever its source, however, a highly cohesive group is one in which members are highly attracted to remain in the group; a group having low cohesiveness is one in which the members are minimally attracted to the group.

Cohesiveness is related to normative pressures in a rather straight-forward way: the more cohesive the group, the greater the normative pressures (Festinger et al., 1950, provide a classic study of this effect). When we focus on an individual member of the group, the same relationship holds; the more attracted a particular member is to his or her group, the more that person will be responsive to normative pressures. Essentially, the more cohesive the group, the more its members are attracted to their membership and want the group to remain together as a group; under these conditions, members give and receive more pressure to follow group norms than do less cohesive groups. In the latter groups, with minimal attraction to membership and little concern for the group as a whole, there is little pressure either given or received to follow group norms.

Combining both relevance and cohesiveness, we would expect groups that are highly cohesive to bring the greatest normative pressures to bear on members for issues that are most relevant and central to the group's functioning. The combination of high cohesiveness and high relevance should produce the greatest pressures; the combination of low cohesiveness and low relevance should produce the least pressure for normative conformity. Often, what seems to be chaotic and confused group functioning and little coordination among the members reflects this very condition of low cohesiveness and low relevance. Research reported by Schachter (1951) has provided some valuable support for the joint effects of relevance and cohesiveness; other investigators have substantially confirmed the connection between a group's level of cohesiveness and the pressures on members to follow group norms (Cartwright & Zander, 1968, provide a useful discussion of some of this work).

THE IMPORTANCE OF UNDERSTANDING GROUP NORMS

Implied throughout our discussion of group norms and normative pressures are reasons why the student of group process would benefit from a knowledge of these concepts. Let us, however, confront the practical issue more directly. Several writers about group process help sharpen our discussion of the practical issues involved.

Lewin's Analysis

In Chapter 1, we introduced some of Lewin's ideas about the role of group processes in behavior maintenance and change. His analysis indicates that a group's norms and standards are *the* critical element in both maintaining an individual's existing behaviors and attitudes and in providing the context for changing them. To understand an individual's health practices, for example, we need to understand the norms of the groups to which that individual belongs or to which he or she aspires to belong (i.e., the person's reference groups). Furthermore, to implement a program of change in that individual's health practices, we would have to effect a change in the norms of those same groups or provide the individual with group contexts whose norms support a more desirable set of health practices. In other words, we can neither understand an individual's existing behaviors and attitudes nor hope to change them without an understanding of the normative processes that are involved.

Argyris's Analysis

While we attach the name of Argyris to this perspective, many others have reached a similar conclusion: often it is the norms of groups that work to prevent the group's effectiveness. Thus, to increase group effectiveness, diagnosing normative patterns and working to change them (Lieberman et al., 1973) is often required. Argyris bases his conclusions on the results of a large-scale investigation of actual problem-solving and decision-making groups in business and industry, the government, universities, and other types of organizations (Argyris, 1969, 1975, 1976; Argyris & Schon, 1974). His data suggested that the dominant pattern of norms that characterized most of these groups (he referred to this as Pattern A) involved: (a) being generally closed to other members' ideas but especially their feelings; (b) being generally distrustful of others; (c) refusing to experiment with alternative ideas or ways of doing things; (d) generally going along with existing norms, valuing conformity to these norms, and trying not to rock the boat. Let us quote Argyris's conclusions about groups characterized by this normative pattern:

> The consequences of Pattern A behavior were relatively ineffective interpersonal relationships and ineffective problem solving of task issues that were important and loaded with feelings. When solutions were achieved, they did not tend to be lasting ones. The problems therefore seemed to recur continually. Finally, members seemed to be blind to the negative impact that they tended to have on others (partially because it violated the norms to give such feedback); they were accurately aware of the impact others have upon them, but careful not to communicate this impact openly or directly. (1969, pp. 898-899)

In that Pattern A seems to predominate in the groups that Argyris has studied and clearly to predominate in most groups of health professionals, the group process practitioner faces a real challenge to his or her practice. What we have noted is that a group's norms can thwart effective group practice; and that the typical normative pattern is one that generally produces ineffective problem-solving. The practitioner must therefore work to evaluate and change group norms in order to have any hope for accomplishing effective group process; and this is nowhere more true than in the health professions.

The health team dealing with the Watts family is a good case in point. If it were to function according to the Pattern A description, then we would expect to find the following things occur:

1. Each specialist on the team would push his or her own point of view and generally be closed to hearing or responding to the views and ideas of other members.

2. Feelings concerning the way the group was functioning or the effective-ness of its treatment plan would never be openly expressed or examined; therefore people on the team would never really know how anyone else felt about what they were supposedly doing together.

3. Team members would act in generally distrustful ways toward one another; they would not reveal ideas and opinions to others if they felt that they would not gain acceptance; they would be wary of one another, and act in polite but distant ways.

4. The possibilities for engaging in innovative treatment plans would be minimized because members felt it was neither appropriate nor wise to experiment with new ideas; the tendency would be for the team to con-tinue to tread the old pathways and not venture into anything new or different.

5. Members would most highly value conforming with existing group norms; in particular, they would be likely to value going along with the medical doctor who heads the team, not wishing to seriously question or challenge his or her ideas, seeing any such challenges as rocking the boat.

It is highly doubtful that a group governed by such norms could function effectively as a team to provide excellent care to Mrs. Watts and her family. To function effectively, this team would have to examine the norms that mem-bers had created together and work toward restructuring those very norms that thwart effective team practice. While this is not an easy process, it is a realistic and possible process; it is one of which the practitioner must be mindful, especially as team practice becomes increasingly a model for health care.

Groupthink and the Conflict Perspective

Based on his examination of high-level governmental decision-making groups, Janis (1973) introduced the term *groupthink* to describe a normative pattern similar in many respects to Argyris' s Pattern A. Groupthink refers to the tendency within many groups to eschew conflict and adopt a norma-tive pattern in which the good group member is loyal to the group's leader and other members, never really challenging or seriously doubting the leader's or the group's wisdom in matters of decision-making. Groupthink, like Pattern A norms, typically leads to ineffective group functioning. Alter-natives are never seriously considered by the group; members fear that to bring up a different possibility is to openly challenge the serene loyalty that is normatively demanded. Members follow groupthink norms, refusing to provide the kinds of seriously probing questions that all decision-making groups need in developing and testing out their proposals before enacting them as policy.

Researchers, such as Maier and his several colleagues, have provided further perspective on this important function; effective group problem-solving derives from encouraging openness and conflict within the group rather than from a normative pattern that discourages any open exchange of ideas and points of view (see Maier, 1970). Maier's research data suggest that both leadership style and group norms that converge around conflict avoidance hinder effective group problem-solving. We will consider this issue of leadership style in Chapter 12. The normative picture is what concerns us at this point. Clearly, if some degree of conflict of ideas is necessary to effective group problem-solving and if excessive loyalty thwarts the introduction of challenges to the existing decisions and alternatives (as with Pattern A or groupthink), then groups characterized by these norms and normative pressures will not be as effective as groups with different norms.

The intimate connection between a group's norms and its effectiveness is sufficiently great to warrant our concern with norms and normative pressures as a matter of urgent practicality. To be able to recognize a group's normative status is important to any student of group process or for that matter, any individuals for whom group process enters as a significant component of their practice.

SUMMARY AND CONCLUSIONS

Group norms refer to shared standards for behavior, attitudes, and perception that characterize all kinds of group. The existence of norms gives rise to pressures on members to follow these norms. These pressures vary as a function of the relevance of the norms to the purposes of the group and the cohesiveness of the group. Norms serve task, maintenance, and social reality functions. The analysis of a group's norms and normative pressures is vital to an understanding of group process. Much of what goes on in groups involves the development and transformation of norms and the processes involved in maintaining members' conformity to norms. It is virtually impossible to comprehend individual behavior in a group without an understanding of group norms and how these norms influence members' conceptions of themselves and their daily practice. The intimate connection between a group's effectiveness and its pattern of norms demands that we understand norms and normative pressures if our interest lies in working more effectively in and with groups.

6

Group Development

*M*uch of our understanding of groups tends to be like snapshots—still photographs taken at one moment and frozen in time. Thus, we fail to see the progression over time that characterizes all human relationships, including the manner through which groups grow and change. We are accustomed to thinking in developmental terms when we deal with individuals. We know, for example that the patterns of behavior we see in the infant and toddler will, in time, give way to those of childhood and then adolescence. At times, it must seem that adolescence will last forever, whereas it actually soon yields to another stage of life involving yet other tasks and an agenda moving towards adulthood and maturity. Is it possible, then, to view groups developmentally as well? And, if so, what would group development look like?

There have been several efforts to examine group development and to provide helpful terms to describe the phases or stages that a group might pass through over time. The main point to keep in mind when considering the various approaches, is that each is an attempt to help us understand that the ways in which groups function when they begin can significantly change over time, often following discernible stages. One helpful quality that developmental analysis can provide, quite simply, is patience. In light of our knowledge of group development, we may be able to guide our groups through some of the more difficult times.

BALES

Bales was especially interested in understanding the small work group that was given a specific problem to solve and a somewhat limited time in which to accomplish a solution. His observations of the patterning of interaction led him to conclude that groups pass through three critical developmental stages, each of which focuses on a specific question (Bales, 1955, 1955b).

ORIENTATION ASKS: "What is the problem?"
EVALUATION ASKS: "How do we feel about it?"
CONTROL ASKS: "What should we do about it?"

To speak of these three as developmental stages is to suggest that whenever a group comes together to deal with a problem, it must confront each of these issues in turn, and answer each of these questions in turn, in order to move toward a solution.

Let us be clear about this matter. One group member may reverse the ordering, trying first to deal with the issue of control even before the problem has been clarified. Another may focus on evaluative issues before considering the dimensions of the task at hand. In other words, this model of development calls our attention to a stagewise developmental sequence that *in general* will characterize successful problem-solving in groups. Individuals may wish to skip stages, but in due time the group will have to return to deal with the prior issues.

In this respect, this developmental model for groups has its parallel in developmental models of individual growth. Adolescents, for example, may wish to rush headlong into the issues of the adult world and bypass those of their own age; yet in time, those earlier issues will have to be dealt with. For example, adolescents may wish to move into an intimate, long-term relationship with another person before they have satisfactorily confronted the prior issues of identity. A safe bet is that the fling at intimacy will not succeed until they make some headway in negotiating the prior issues of identity.

Much the same idea can be applied to Bales's three stages of group development. To attend to stage two issues of evaluation or stage three matters of control before even orienting the group to the nature and dimensions of the problem will only delay dealing with the prior matter. As we will see in the chapter on leadership, a group leader, aware of these stages of development and skillful in diagnosing a group's present location along this sequence, can prove helpful in redirecting a group and thereby facilitating its development. That is, the leader can help the group pass through its normal developmental sequence by returning members to earlier issues if they deal with later issues out of their proper sequence. The member who wishes to focus on control when the problem has not yet even been clarified can be helpfully redirected to begin with first things first.

TUCKMAN

In 1965, Bruce Tuckman attempted to synthesize the literature on group development. He suggested that four main developmental stages characterized most of the theories he reviewed. He further noted that developmental issues could be examined separately for the interpersonal and for the task areas for each stage. As with Bales's and the other theories we examine, it makes sense to consider each stage to be *an issue* that the group must consider and resolve in some manner in order to move forward to the next stage.

Stage I: Forming

INTERPERSONAL ISSUES: This is similar to Bales's idea of orientation. All groups must initially deal with the issues of coming together, of forming a group. These include trying to get to know the members and seeking leadership and direction.

TASK ISSUES: During the forming phase, the main concern in the task arena involves defining the purpose of the group, its goals, who has what kinds of knowledge and information pertinent to those goals, and so on.

Stage II: Storming

INTERPERSONAL ISSUES: Storming involves a period of tension and conflict; subgroups begin to form based on mutual interests or similarity in points of view; subgroups clashing with one another produce conflicts and disagreements within the group.

TASK ISSUES: Storming in the task area emphasizes substantive disagreements regarding the best way to proceed, disagreements about leadership and control, and so forth.

Stage III: Norming

INTERPERSONAL ISSUES: During this phase, the group has weathered conflicts and seeks now to develop norms conducive to group cohesion and working together effectively.

TASK ISSUES: At this stage, the task issues begin to deal with sharing different interpretations and perspectives about the task; seeking to reach a consensus and developing cooperative working relationships.

Stage IV: Performing

INTERPERSONAL ISSUES: Now that the group has moved through its other phases, it is ready to work together as an effective unit. Interpersonal issues focus on the best ways to establish functional role relationships among members so that time spent together is productive.

TASK ISSUES: The group spends this phase seeking effective and acceptable solutions to the task issue that brought them together as a group in the first place.

It is important for the student of group process to reflect for a moment on the stages that Tuckman has summarized. In particular, the presence of a stage of conflict is important to consider. In this view, conflict and disagreement over task and personal issues is seen to be a normal developmental stage that all groups must pass through before they can get down to the business of doing the actual job for which they have convened. Conflict, therefore, is not inevitably destructive nor a symptom of a faulty group; in fact, it is something to deal with and to build upon.

A group that jumped from forming to norming, for example, refusing to deal with the underlying disagreements that exist whenever persons are convened to work together, might initially appear happy, harmonious, and in agreement. Yet one would suspect that its underlying disagreements and conflicts, never having been confronted directly in the storming phase, would emerge in many subtle and not-too-subtle ways perhaps to sabotage the group's effectiveness in performing.

The group leader would do well to consider these normal stages of development. In particular, it is useful to hypothesize that the absence of a storming period does not mean, "I've got a good group." It may mean that something is inhibiting members' expression of their disagreements; this is not a good sign for the group's long-term work together. Likewise, a group leader would do well not to shudder and abandon all hope should the normal period of storming occur. Needless to say, we are not encouraging the wholesale abandonment of reason to full-fledged storming. We are encouraging persons to consider very carefully the implications of a developmental model of group process in which storming is considered part of the normal growth process and not an aberrant tendency.

SCHUTZ

William Schutz (1960) developed a theory of interpersonal needs, a test to measure those needs, and a conception of group development that built upon both. The theory is similar in many respects to the psychoanalytic models that parented it. Schutz suggests that all persons have what he terms interpersonal needs; these are needs that can be satisfied only by and with others. They are said to be three in number: *inclusion, control,* and *affection.* Each involves a particular issue or set of related issues. Inclusion involves the issue of belonging, of being in or of being out, of bringing others in or excluding and rejecting others. Control involves issues of authority, of dominance, and of submission. Affection involves issues of intimacy, of closeness, of caring, of disliking, of distancing.

Schutz's developmental theory argued that these three interpersonal needs, in the I-C-A order (inclusion-control-affection) describe the developmental stages that groups pass through in coming together and working together. He further suggested a point that the other theories we have considered have ignored—namely, a developmental sequence for the *termination* of a group. Here, he indicated that the termination order reverses the original sequence and takes the form of A-C-I. Let us briefly examine each of these in turn.

Forming

The I-C-A developmental pattern suggests two important matters: first, the critical issues that groups must confront; second, the ordering with which these issues are faced. In this respect, Schutz's concept of group development is similar to all concepts of development: a set of critical issues or critical stages is introduced and an ordering to these is provided.

Inclusion

The first issue confronting a group involves *inclusion*. Somewhat similar to both orientation and forming, inclusion focuses on the issues of membership and commitment. It is said that groups must consider who the members really are, who is committed to the group, who rightfully belongs, and who is present but not a true member.

It might sound strange to speak about inclusion as an issue for most work groups; after all, the membership is assigned by the work setting and thus presumably everyone who is said to be a member of the group or the team is a member. Thus, supposedly the inclusion issue is handled formally and thereby, in this view, surely cannot be an issue for the group. On the contrary, inclusion remains an issue to be considered by the group even when a formal assignment of members has been made. Inclusion also deals with the more subtle kinds of in-out relationships, especially those involving different levels of commitment to and involvement with the group as a group. Formal and non-voluntary work groups are especially prone to inclusion issues; after all, people were simply thrown together and implicitly told to be a group. Yet this is not sufficient to make them a group until they can focus on the inclusion issues, especially the more subtle meanings of membership and commitment.

Control and Affection

The issue of control, the next in the developmental sequence according to Schutz, focuses on the critical theme of authority, dependence, and autonomy.

Schutz suggests that issues of control and relationships with authority precede issues of affection and intimacy. It is as though one cannot begin to relate on a basis of equality within the group, to explore more fully with one another the various kinds of attractions and repulsions that exist, until one has first dealt with matters of control. These tend to differentiate and often stratify members into the more and less powerful or influential; and until this is dealt with, other aspects of member relationships, involving attraction and intimacy, cannot be confronted as directly.

Terminating

In terminating, Schutz suggests that groups pass through these same stages but in a reverse order. Thus, the first issues that come before the group as they head toward their termination involve the bonds of attraction that were involved. Next, issues of control are considered; and finally, inclusion, as the group or the relationship ends.

Keep in mind that these issues will not always be as openly expressed as our description suggests. As we observe a group in action, we will not inevitably witness persons speaking directly about "inclusion" or "control" or "affection." What we must learn to do, therefore, is to inquire and to probe beyond the surface manifestations and content that is directly discussed; we must look for symptoms of these underlying themes and issues and ask ourselves if an understanding of such issues helps us better comprehend what is taking place in the group.

An Example

When a group convenes for the first time and we observe its interaction, the word "inclusion" will probably never be spoken; people may not discuss commitment to the group, who is in and who is out, what it means to be a member of this group, and so forth. People may only talk about job-related issues, concerning a particular patient, for example. There will be different rates of participation in the discussion; there may even be some disagreements; certain persons may seen more involved and interested in the discussion, while others may seem more withdrawn into their personal issues, or bored with what is happening, or talking on seemingly irrelevant matters.

If we study this group with the Schutz scheme in mind, inclusion is likely to be discovered as an underlying issue that will help explain many aspects of what we observe; members will express in various ways (not always explicitly) their different needs for being included, their fears about being a member and committed to the group and to others, their desires to bring in or include others, and so forth.

We would suspect that inclusion issues are relevant and are being dealt with in often subtle and indirect ways. We would also expect that individual differences in commitment to the group, as evidenced for example in different amounts of participation and concern for the group's welfare, are important matters for the group to deal with openly and directly before such inclusion issues become hindrances to the group's working effectiveness. A leader of this group would use his or her theoretical sensitivities to this possibility to help facilitate the group's dealing with whatever issues and conflicts arise over, in this instance, inclusion and commitment. Members' attention may even have to be focused on their differences in apparent contribution and involvement in the group. Do these reflect differences in commitment to the group? Are these differences proving troublesome to the group's functioning?

Basically, the developmental theory can be used as a tool to help guide our understanding and our intervention; it provides us with a useful interpretative framework for putting together what would otherwise be discrete bits and pieces of observed information. But, most importantly, the developmental models generate hypotheses about what may be taking place; thereby they help us work more effectively with the group.

Of course, these are just hypotheses, tentative proposals and interpretations rather than facts carved in granite. Thus we must remain open to the possibility that what the theory suggests is happening or should be happening, may not be. But without a theoretical tool, we could not even formulate clear hypotheses about what was taking place and thus not even be able to prove ourselves to be wrong about what we see. A good theory, therefore, lets us know when we are wrong as well as helping to guide us in more correct directions.

LUFT

While Joseph Luft's ideas are not restricted to group development, they do offer us another set of concepts useful for understanding certain developmental processes within groups (Luft, 1970). Luft's contention is that interpersonal relationships can be charted in terms of the degree to which one's self and others are aware of one's self. Four different possibilities have been defined as follows:

OPEN AREA: This includes material that is both known to the self and available to be known to others. For example, both Jane and I know that Jane is a nurse.

BLIND AREA: This includes material that is not known to the self, but which others are able to discern. For example, Barry is not aware that his abrupt, somewhat arrogant manner of talking down to his patients is upsetting to them, but most people who work with him are well aware of these effects.

HIDDEN AREA: This includes material that is known to the self but hidden from others' knowledge. For example, Roseanne is aware that she is very worried about getting AIDS from some of her patients, but hides this fear from her co-workers, who do not seem to be as troubled by this as she is.

UNKNOWN AREA: This includes material that is unknown both to self and the others. We assume that there are aspects of all of us that we and others are currently unaware of, but that could come into awareness at some point.

Regarding issues of group development, Luft posits that the open area will grow larger, the blind area will become smaller and the hidden area will have less impact in groups that work effectively together. In effect, Luft is suggesting that through working together over time, people will become more open to one another, learn more about each other's ideas and skills, and increase the open area. In turn, as that area grows, the area that we try to defend from others' knowledge—the hidden area—should begin to contract, or at least its impact on our interaction should be reduced. Finally, the blind area, encompassing things about ourselves we currently do not know but of which others are aware, should decrease as we and they become better able to share more of our genuine feelings and attitudes.

BENNIS AND SHEPARD

Luft's ideas lead naturally to the final theory of development we will consider, proposed several years ago by Bennis and Shepard (1956). Consensual validation, the final phase they suggest to be the goal toward which all effective groups should be striving is of pertinence to us. In other words, their developmental theory offers us a glimpse of the end state of good group development, reminiscent, in certain respects, of the ideals conveyed in Luft's own analysis. Let us examine the several key features of this idealized goal of effective group development, considering it to be just that, an ideal toward which groups can strive, but rarely reach.

The final state is termed *consensual validation* and in it:

1. Members have learned to accept one another's differences without labeling those differences as either "good" or "bad." This is considered a significant advance and sign of growth in any group: when people have moved far enough along in their working relationship that the initial rejections of one another's ideas or abilities is replaced with an openness and acceptance of the things that make one person different from another.

2. Conflicts and disagreements continue to exist within the group, but tend to focus primarily around substantive issues rather than hidden, emotional concerns. It is important to realize once again that a good group is not characterized by the absence of conflict or disagreement; rather a good group has conflicts that are based on genuine differences in people's beliefs, attitudes, points of view, and so forth. People can talk about these differences and negotiate working agreements rather than engaging in conflicts that remain boiling just beneath the surface and continue to capture people's attention and drain their energy.

3. Consensus is reached through rational discussion and reasoned negotiation rather than through compulsive attempts to wring uniformity—as a test of loyalty or obedience—from the group. It is recognized that too many groups insist on members' blind obedience or loyalty, assuming that any disagreements within the group are akin to a betrayal. Under these conditions, consensus is hardly an ideal. The ideal refers to a consensus achieved by bridging the differences that exist on the basis of a rational discussion and negotiation among equal participants.

4. Stereotyped expectations about one another are replaced with more realistic expectations that stem from a genuine understanding of one another.
Once again, Bennis and Shepard present us with an ideal, not necessarily
with what one typically finds in groups. When the ideal is reached, people
relate to one another on a more personal basis due to their mutual understanding of how each person in the group thinks and acts. Stereotypes
about one another too often rule both the early and the later life of a group:
people continue to interact with cardboard figures—stereotypes—rather
than real people.

Remember, these four elements describe the ideal goals toward which
groups should be striving as they develop rather than the reality that most
groups actually achieve. This realization might help lessen the frustration
that many will experience when comparing their own current groups with
this ideal. The ideal of consensual validation marks a standard and a serious
challenge to all group members and leaders alike.

SUMMARY AND CONCLUSIONS

An analysis of theories of group development provides us with additional
tools by which to understand and to intervene effectively in group process.
All developmental theories offer us two related points: (1) each outlines the
critical issues that are said to confront all groups; (2) each outlines the particular sequence or order in which these issues are said to occur. Not surprisingly, whatever the particular persuasion of the theory, most approaches
suggest that issues centering around authority and leadership on the one
hand and around member-to-member relationships on the other will prove
central to all groups. And most theories locate these developmentally in the
sequence: authority issues precede peer relations.

It is important to keep in mind that all developmental concepts have
an ordering that repeats itself throughout the life of the group. That is, a
particular developmental stage or issue is never fully completed for all time;
rather, as circumstances change, the same developmental issue may crop up
again and again. For example, using Bales's analysis, problems of orientation will present themselves again within the life of the group whenever the
task changes or whenever a new problem emerges to be dealt with. Or, to
use Schutz's model, inclusion will be an issue whenever members change
(some old members leave and new members enter the group) or even when
the task itself changes and a new kind of group formation may be necessary.

In light of the preceding, it is best to think of a developmental *spiral*
rather than a developmental line. A line suggests a beginning and a definite
end. A spiral suggests a continuing turn around and around similar issues;
it also suggests progress and growth at the same time. Thus, the issues of
orientation or of inclusion, for example, will appear again within the life

history of a group; but their second appearance will not be the same as their first; nor will the third be exactly the same as the second, and so forth. In other words, the model of a spiral suggests similar issues that are dealt with in somewhat different ways each time they reappear within a group.

The lessons of group development are important for the group leader. Often, the only sense that can be made out of a given kind of interaction is found through an understanding of the developmental issue that is involved. Furthermore, leader interventions require an understanding of normal group development. Timing of interventions is something that is especially linked to an understanding of development. To push a group too fast toward a later stage when it is still caught up in early-stage issues, for example, does the same to the group that it can do to the individual: i.e., it confuses, leads to resistance, creates frustration, and produces needless tension and conflict.

III

Theoretical Perspectives

*W*hile some people anticipate boredom when the word *theory* is mentioned, we believe that the advice once given by a prominent social psychologist, Kurt Lewin, continues to be true: There is nothing as practical as a good theory. We are well aware that there are many theories regarding group process, some large and all-encompassing, some small and narrowly focused. Having surveyed the majority of these, we have chosen three major theoretical perspectives to present. Chapter 7 introduces us to systems theory, better thought of as a way of thinking than a formal theory. Our purpose in this chapter is to help lay the foundation for this rather unique and currently important way of trying to understand group process.

Chapter 8 introduces the concept of unconscious processes, an idea with which we are generally familiar when dealing with individuals, but one which may initially appear to be rather unusual when referring to groups. We hope to provide a convincing case for both the meaningfulness of considering groups to have an unconscious life and for examining some of those unconscious dimensions.

In Chapter 9, we introduce the important topic of intergroup relations. We argue that our lives are increasingly influenced by group memberships and that an understanding of the role of these memberships—the basis for intergroup dynamics—is therefore important.

7

Systems Theory

Consider the following situation that outlines certain aspects of the U.S. health-care system in terms of a means—ends analysis:

THE ENDS

Most people would agree that the highly valued goals or ends of an ideal health-care system would be (a) to provide access to all persons in the society who need services, (b) to provide the highest possible quality services and (c) to accomplish all of this at the lowest costs possible (Aday, 1987; Kiesler & Morton, 1988).

THE MEANS

Many people would also agree that among the factors most likely to lead to those valued goals, the following three are central: (a) Consumers should have freedom of choice in selecting their health-care providers; (b) providers (especially physicians) should be autonomous agents in charge of deciding the best approach in treating their patients and in setting the appropriate fees to charge for their services; (c) a freemarket (i.e., unregulated) health-care system in which independent entrepreneurs compete with one another to provide services will work best for all concerned.

SOME OUTCOMES

As the means are put into operation, certain outcomes begin to take shape that undermine the attainment of the very ends that those means were presumably meant to accomplish.

1. The fee-for-service system operates as an incentive to order and perform many tests, in that the more services provided, the more money can be made by the providers.

2. In an increasingly litigiousness society, increased testing also stems from a concern to protect one's self against allegations of improper practice.

3. The reimbursement system, by reimbursing providers on the basis of the prevailing fees for services in a given community, encourages providers to establish their practices in higher priced rather than in poor or rural areas, thereby undermining access to health care for many segments of the population.

4. By reimbursing providers on the basis of their record of previous charges, providers are encouraged to push charges even higher in order to keep the historical profile on which current charges are paid as high as possible.

What has occurred, in effect, is a situation in which two of the three goals—access and cost-containment—have clearly been undermined by the manner in which the system originally established to achieve those goals operates. The third goal, high-quality health care, may itself be jeopardized by the manner in which the system functions.

In response to these failures, the government, employers, and insurers have sought to intervene by transforming consumer choice, professional sovereignty, and freemarket competition, thereby challenging the foundations on which the entire U.S. system of services, including health care, rests.

THE LESSONS LEARNED

Two qualities in the preceding illustration are important to consider from a systems perspective. First, as we have seen, the elements of the system designed to achieve certain goals actually had the opposite effect as the system operated over time. A system designed to provide access, autonomy, low cost, and high quality care therefore thwarted ready access to millions of consumers, undermined autonomy, produced increasingly higher costs for care, and possibly reduced the quality of care or, at minimum, raised serious questions about that quality.

Although the functioning of all systems does not invariably invert the system's fundamental qualities, the example does prove a point that holds true for all systems—that one cannot readily predict the outcome of a system from a knowledge of the initial conditions of the system. In this respect, systems theory differs from most other theories that attempt to understand group and organizational processes.

The example rather clearly demonstrates the second point, that each element in the overall picture of the health-care system is related, very closely and interdependently, with every other element in the system. In other words, the parts of the system do not stand alone, nor do they operate independently of one another. The elements of any system affect, and are affected by, the other elements in the system. For example, the way in which hospitals are paid (element #1) helps increase the number of services performed (element #2), which leads to higher overall medical costs (element #3), which in turn, leads those footing the bill to seek the containment of costs (element #4), and so on.

Once we enter the world of systems theory, we are no longer able to speak simply of elements or parts existing separately from one another. Relationships and interconnections are central to any systems analysis. The following are some of the essentials of systems theory. Much of our analysis is based on several key sources that discuss this issue in detail (Bateson, 1972; Bertalanffy, 1950; Miller, 1965; Scott, 1981; Tubbs, 1978; Watzlawick, et al., 1967).

THE SYSTEMS MODEL

Efforts to understand something as complex as human behavior, both individual and group, have turned to several guiding frameworks derived from other sciences. Early physical theory, especially the Newtonian world view, offered us a machinelike analysis of nature that was all too easily transferred to the realm of the human. Human life was considered to be like a giant machine with mechanical links and connections exercising their direct and clocklike control over the person and society. In time, the Newtonian concepts in physics gave way to a less neat mechanical view of the physical world. New models were introduced to enrich the knowledge of human behavior.

Many of these new models turned away from the physical sciences' perspective and turned to the view emerging within the life sciences. The organic model of nature, derived largely from the study of living biological systems, offered an attractive way of understanding human life.

When we adopt an organic or biological metaphor, we consider the subject of interest to us (e.g., the health-care system; group process) as though it was a living system. As we know, living systems (also called open as contrasted with closed systems) are composed of elements that function together and that engage in an exchange relationship with their environments. The human body is such a system: its parts consist of several subsystems that are interrelated (i.e., interact with one another) and that function together to achieve a balance or an equilibrium both internally and in exchanges with the surrounding environment.

The very concept of system suggests parts that hang together, that work together, and are interdependent even though specialized in their function. Thus, if a group is said to function like a system, the parts (i.e., members) behave differently together than when not part of that system we call the group. Likewise, if we consider a group as a system, we are concerned with the ways in which that system achieves a steady state or equilibrium through its exchanges both with its internal environment (i.e., its member-to-member relations) and its external environment (i.e., the groups' relations with other groups, its designated task, the organization within which it functions, and so forth).

The organic metaphor teaches us that in order to understand the activities of the parts, we must first understand their location and function within an equilibrium-maintaining system. For example, we might understand the failure of a kidney to perform its proper function by viewing it within the context of the whole living body of which it is a part. That is, the demand on the kidney was increased leading to its failure because another subsystem of the body failed to function properly. In a similar way, we attempt to understand the behavior of any single group member by viewing it within the context of the living system (the group) of which it was a part. Let us now examine several important characteristics of all systems.

Elements

A system contains elements or parts. A group, for example, contains individuals who are its members. A family contains individuals who are its members. An organization (e.g., a hospital) contains individuals and units that are its elements. Even something as vast as the nation's method of offering and financing health care, as we have seen, can function as a system containing quite large and complex elements. An element in one system can be considered an entire system from another perspective. Thus, for example, the individual is an element in a group; yet from the perspective of bodily functioning, the individual is the system and the body parts are the elements. Or, from still another perspective, the circulatory system is the "system" and the elements involve heart, lungs, blood, and so forth. In our opening example, the hospital, one element in the nation's overall health-care system, is in itself a complex system, containing many elements.

Interdependence

The elements of any system are joined together by a relationship of interdependence. Thus, whatever happens to one element in the system has consequences for other elements of that same system. The actions of one group member, for example, affect the actions of other members of the group. Whenever elements are joined into a system, their behavior is no longer independent. The behavior of any one part is thereby intimately linked to the behavior of all the other parts. And, as we have already observed, the health-care system as a whole clearly reveals this feature of interdependence.

Wholistic Functioning

The interdependent elements of a system are organized into a whole and function together as a whole. Furthermore, the whole has properties that no element necessarily has. And these properties or characteristics of the whole affect the behavior of each of the elements of the system. Thus, a group has characteristics that no member of the group possesses. It is commonly noted that the whole is different than the mere sum of its parts. A group can be aggressive and combative, for example, whereas members in isolation from one another are more docile and less aggressive. There is something about their coming together into a group that creates aggression as a property of their group as a whole. By noting that properties of the whole affect the behavior of the elements, we are suggesting that members will take on characteristics in one system that are aspects of that system; in another system, they may behave very differently. The adolescent, for example, may be very friendly and open at home but aggressive and hostile or withdrawn and unfriendly at school. Parts in different systems are not the same.

Once again, the opening example illustrates the wholistic functioning of systems. It is possible, for example, to speak of the overall systems of health-care in Great Britain, Canada, or France. In each case, we treat an entire system as a whole, examining how the U.S. system as a whole functions as compared to other national systems of health care, which, as Starr (1982), among others, points out, operate in a very different manner.

Causal Analysis

Given the preceding information, we can see that in order to understand the behavior of any element of a system, we must first understand its location within the system. That is, an element is not the same when it is in a different system. To the teachers, the 14-year-old girl may be aggressive or excessively withdrawn; to her parents, she is warm, open, and friendly. Which one is the true person? Both. She can only be understood in the context of school or home. Likewise, when we try to understand the behavior of any member of a group, we must locate our analysis in the ongoing context of that group. Our causal analysis—that is, how we go about understanding the causes of behavior—requires our consideration of the system or context within which the particular element is functioning.

In the opening example, we pointed out the special kind of causal analysis that appears in systems theory. We noted that the final state—the outcome—of the system's operation could not be predicted from a knowledge of its initial conditions—the input. Recall that in the example the initial conditions were presumably designed to achieve several goals: low-cost, high-quality health-care for everyone; freedom of choice for the consumer; autonomy for the provider. The outcomes, however inverted all of these, as the system created conditions that undermined the realization of the very initial conditions put into it.

In the usual framework of causal analysis, a linear view of cause and effect is maintained, whereby X is said to be the cause and Y, the effect. X and Y are in a linear relationship such that whenever X appears, Y will also appear. When we have a linear condition of this sort we can predict the later state (e.g., Y) from a knowledge of the initial condition (e.g., X). Once we enter the world of system's theory, however, it is clear that all such bets must be called off. What happens later cannot readily be known from knowledge of those initial conditions or inputs. Will Y result when X is input? We cannot say. And, as we have seen, though we may wish X to cause Y, X may set in motion a series of events that, over time, produce the obverse of Y!

Equilibrium

One of the major properties of all systems is their tendency to seek some point of balance or equilibrium. This property calls our attention to the ways in which systems restore homeostasis whenever events disturb the ongoing state of balance. Most systems with which we deal are termed *open systems*. An open system is one that receives inputs from its environment and sends outputs back into the environment. Open systems are in an exchange with their environment; they are thereby open to having their equilibrium upset. In the living organism, for example, there is an exchange in which oxygen and other nutrients come in and waste products go out. Balance between this input and outflow is a characteristic of such a system. When that balance is upset, illness results.

In a similar manner, when we consider the group to be an open system that seeks equilibrium, we ask about the mechanism by which that group maintains its equilibrium in the face of changing environmental inputs. A family, for example, may have achieved an excellent equilibrium as long as the wife remains at home and does household chores, the husband is away at work, and the children remain young and in school. That equilibrium can be upset, however, by any number of inputs: e.g., the wife gets a job; the children get older and leave home; the husband loses or changes his job; a severe illness strikes one member of the family; and so on.

Basically, any change threatens the stability of a system and thus is resisted. We can learn a great deal about how a system (e.g., a group or a family) maintains its equilibrium by observing what happens when changes are instituted. In psychiatric practice, for example, it has long been observed that as the identified "sick" member is brought into treatment and threatens to get better, other members of the family may begin to get worse. In other words, the family's equilibrium around the "sick member" is threatened by that person's return to health; this then triggers new mechanisms of adjustment designed to retain the entire system in a state of equilibrium. These mechanisms may take the form of withdrawing the sick member from therapy so as to return him or her to the "sick status," or by another member's developing symptoms of illness, or even by the failure of the equilibrium to be restored and the family's dissolution.

The kind of equilibrium that exists in the opening illustration is not quite the same sort observed in these other examples. Indeed, the health-care system in the illustration is seen to be a system that is out of control, not one in a state of equilibrium. The example illustrates a system that is spiraling above a point of equilibrium rather than one that returns, like a thermostat, to a balance point. This then brings us to the next feature of a system's analysis, feedback.

Feedback

The information that is fed into a system (either from the outside or from within) which keeps it on course is referred to as feedback. The information, for example, that a thermostat receives regarding room temperature helps adjust the control mechanism directing the heat to be turned off or turned on. Feedback refers to any information that helps steer, guide, or direct the behavior of a system or its elements. The equilibrium of a system is maintained by virtue of feedback mechanisms. In a group, for example, the leader may help steer the group by providing it feedback regarding its present state with respect to its goals.

A thermostat is controlled by *negative* feedback. *Positive* feedback, by contrast, amplifies the effects of a process and thus leads a system to move beyond equilibrium. This describes the operation of the overall health-care system of the opening example. We noted that the ways in which reimbursement for services is provided, for example, proves to be an incentive for amplifying the tendency to provide more and more costly services rather than for diminishing the number or complexity of services. Feedback relations, in this case, do not produce a steady state based on negative feedback, but involve the amplifying effects of positive feedback.

One can also see the effects of positive feedback occurring in a group when, for example, deep feelings of anger are aroused and one person's accusations trigger another's equally aggressive response, in turn triggering even more intense exchanges of negative feelings. All of this begins to spiral out of control unless some kind of equilibrium-restoring intervention is initiated or until the group breaks apart.

A WAY OF THINKING

The systems perspective offers us a way of looking at a wide variety of phenomena. It directs attention to certain aspects of reality; it helps organize our experience and provide us with the tools we need for better understanding. When we speak about the group as a system, we are adopting a perspective that emphasizes (a) how structures and relationships emerge within a group; (b) how they grow and develop over time; (c) how they are maintained at a relatively steady or stable state; and (d) how they are transformed or changed. This perspective directs our attention to the ways in which groups deal with their task and maintenance problems, the ways in which members are recruited and socialized into their particular roles, how decisions are made, how conflict and disagreement are handled, how leadership and authority are exercised, how relationships develop and evolve over time. Let us use a concrete example to help further illustrate this perspective.

THE WATTS FAMILY AND SYSTEMS ANALYSIS:
AN EXAMPLE

A team of six health professionals, consisting of a physician, a nurse-specialist, a nutritionist, a physical therapist, a psychologist, and a social worker comprise a rehabilitation team to work with Mrs. Watts and her family throughout Mrs. Watts's colostomy surgery and afterward. Their goal is to draw up a plan that will speed her recovery and improve the quality of her life. Their concern is not only with their patient, Mrs. Watts, but with the entire Watts family. The nurse-specialist is primarily concerned with teaching Mrs. Watts how to deal with her colostomy so she can function in a reasonably normal manner. The nutritionist's concern is with issues of proper diet; the physical therapist focuses on helping Mrs. Watts rebuild her strength; the psychologist works with her and her entire family to help them deal with the various emotional problems that have emerged because of her surgery; the social worker joins the psychologist in this endeavor and in addition is concerned with developing community-wide support services for the Watts family. In working with the entire Watts family, members of the team become aware of a variety of medical and psychological problems other than the colostomy alone. Daughter Amy, for example, has an obesity problem that seems to have been exacerbated by her mother's surgery. Son Tim has been having school problems. Mr. Watts has had difficulty in getting and retaining employment and seems especially resentful of all the extra care, attention, and expenditures that his wife's illness demands.

The Team

A systems perspective could focus on the rehabilitation team and its activities or on the Watts family and its mode of functioning. If the team were the focus of our concern, then we would focus on such questions as: How is information brought together from the several different sources? How are decisions made about the family's treatment and progress? Who interacts with whom on the team? Who seems to be most and who seems to be least influential in this decision-making process? How effective is this team? Are there arrangements that would improve the team's efforts? How does its organization affect its effectiveness? What developments in the team interactions and communications have occurred as the members have worked together over time? How are points of view that differ from the majority opinion handled? How is conflict and disagreement handled?

The Family

Our focus, however, need not be restricted to the team of health professionals; we could focus on the Watts family. Many of the same issues and questions would then be of concern to us: e.g., What pattern of interaction and communication characterizes this family? How are family decisions made? How is conflict handled? In what ways are the medical problems expressed within the family? What is the effect on the family of Mrs. Watts's colostomy?

Basically, we would view the family as a system; thereby, we would come to see that the well-being of any member of the family depends on our ability to deal effectively with the family as a whole. We would try to understand, for example, how the daughter's obesity problem and the son's school problem fit into this family's modes of dealing with its medical problems. That is, we would attempt to understand how the multiple problems facing this family weave themselves into a whole, a fabric with its own characteristics. We would adopt this wholistic focus rather than attending to each problem as though it existed in isolation from other problems within the family. The search for the interdependence of parts with the whole, the search for ways in which functions for the whole family are served by the behaviors and symptoms of the members are critical aspects of a system's perspective.

We can reasonably consider the Watts family as having achieved a state of equilibrium before the diagnosis of cancer in Mrs. Watts. Although we cannot be certain about the aspects that comprise that equilibrium, we can feel fairly confident in assuming that any intact and functioning group (family, in this case) has achieved an equilibrium among its constituent parts. Second, we note that Mrs. Watts's diagnosis of cancer and her eventual surgery upset the family's equilibrium; it changed her relationship to others in the family as the illness took her away from her usual functions and cast these upon other family members. The husband, for example, may have had to take on maintenance chores (e.g., caring for the children and the house) in addition to his regular task activities. Likewise, the children, Amy and Tim, may have been forced to assume greater independence once their mother's function in this regard was lost because of her illness.

If we think of the family in these terms, then our next task is to examine the possible connections between Amy's obesity, Tim's school difficulties, Mr. Watts's employment problems, and Mrs. Watts's illness. We may discover, for example, that Amy's obesity is her way of dealing with the tension she is experiencing by being suddenly cast into the role of "mother," having to take care of the others in her household. Likewise, we may discover that Tim's school problems, especially if their onset correlates with Mrs. Watts's illness, is a reaction on his part to his mother's problems. Mr. Watts's resentment may be reflected through his employment difficulties. Each of these is a real possibility that cannot be discounted as the rehabilitation team confronts the Watts family and attempts to facilitate Mrs. Watts's recovery. Her own recovery can be helped or hampered by the family's attitudes and reactions to her illness.

Interventions designed to deal with any one of these problems must clearly be based upon an analysis of the family's process. Approaching Amy's obesity, for example, without locating it within the matrix of this family's process would not be appropriately responsive to its bases and thus is not likely to be successful. Likewise, Tim's school problems must be seen within the context of the Watts family, as must Mr. Watts's employment difficulties and the course of Mrs. Watts's own recovery. The task that the rehab team faces, therefore, requires that each member work in concert with the others of the team to design the kind of care plan for the entire family that builds upon a recognition and understanding of its group process.

Using Lewin's ideas, we can note that interventions that simply add pressures to one side of the family's process equation are likely only to increase tension, solving little. Like adding to wages without resolving issues of fatigue, placing pressure on one element of the system without reducing pressure in another will only result in greater overall tension. For example, treating Mrs. Watts without treating her entire family is likely only to worsen an already unhealthy equilibrium. The team's responsibility therefore is to assess the total configuration of factors acting on the family attributable to Mrs. Watts's colostomy; and then to work within that broadened conception of "patient."

Group Process and the Health Professional Team

The same kind of process perspective is applicable to the rehabilitation team in our example as well as to its target group, the Watts family. By now it should be obvious that the management of the patient depends on a fine coordination among the participants of the health team. No one of them possesses the key to Mrs. Watts's health; but together, they can bring their varied abilities and skills to bear to promote her health and the well-being of the family. How they function as a team is critical to how well they accomplish their goal of facilitating her recovery.

If we examine the team with a systems perspective, we will be concerned with how it goes about accomplishing its task. In particular, we will be concerned with the ways in which it gathers the diverse kinds of information that are necessary to develop a treatment plan, the ways in which this information is coordinated and a plan proposed, and the ways in which the plan is put into effect. Each member of the team has access to a different view of the patient and her family. How are these different views brought together? How are they coordinated into a treatment plan? How is that plan actually carried out? How is the plan evaluated? How are modifications introduced?

Each of these questions focuses our attention on the ways in which the team goes about its business, the ways it manages itself in the process of managing the patient. Notice that our questions are concerned with *how* the group—the family, the team—functions in carrying out its business. In the example, the business involves the delicate coordination of diverse specialties; our attention is focused on how this coordination is accomplished. We are interested in getting an answer so that we can work to develop a more effective group process. Fundamentally, it is only through our understanding of the process whereby groups function as they conduct their business that we can hope to intervene when necessary to effect an improved process.

In the particular team of our example, we may discover that the expertise of the nutritionist is being ignored by other team members as a treatment plan is developed. Or we may note that the psychologist's perspective is seen to be irrelevant by the physician and nurse-specialist. The team functions, therefore, by avoiding true team behavior: that is, it is a team in name only but not in actual practice. Once we know how it functions, we can be helpful in improving its operation so that it can become more of a team in practice as well as in name.

If medical problems such as those of Mrs. Watts are really family problems as well, if the course of the patient's recovery is dependent on working with the family system, then surely a real team is required. And we cannot intervene with the aim of achieving that reality until we can determine the process by which the team (or group or family) functions in the first place.

SUMMARY AND CONCLUSIONS

This chapter has introduced a way of thinking, termed systems theory, that differs in several important respects from the ways of thinking we typically employ when trying to understand different aspects of human life and experience. Rather than breaking a large and complex whole down into its parts and analyzing those parts in the hope that this will give us an understanding of how the whole works, the systems perspective asks us to look at the whole and to see the parts as being so deeply interconnected with one another that their qualities are shaped by the particular whole in which they exist.

The systems perspective, rather than assuming a direct, linear model of cause and effect, teaches us that so much can take place between input and outcome that one cannot readily predict the latter from a knowledge of the former.

Rather than adopting a strategy of simplification—in which we try to isolate the one or two factors that may account for human behavior—the systems perspective also asks us to complicate our thinking by looking for the entire web of interconnected factors that permeate the system and for the networks of positive and negative feedback that join every part of the system with every other part.

The system analysis introduced in this chapter asks us to reframe the ways we look at groups and organizations, and indeed, even the ways we look at ourselves and other individuals.

8

The Unconscious
Dynamics in Groups

Some students of group process may find this chapter, which deals with the unconscious dynamics of groups, somewhat puzzling; to others, this material may be unsettling; still others may view anything on the unconscious as just another bit of "psychobabble."

To make our position clear from the outset: We have been working with groups for too many years to harbor even the slightest doubt that unconscious factors play an important role in all of our group activities. We hope this chapter will clarify the issue for those who are puzzled, reassure those who may be a bit unsettled, and prove to be informative to those who are skeptical about the importance of the unconscious in group dynamics, as well as all those who work everyday with groups as part of their professional lives.

THE UNCONSCIOUS AND THE GROUP'S
HIDDEN AGENDA

We opened a ten-week lecture-lab course on group process on Tuesday with a brief lecture on the meaning of groups and group membership. We then told the students that on Thursday they would not convene with one of us standing up in front of the room lecturing, but rather as an unstructured group, with neither a leader in charge nor an agenda to direct their time together. Thursday arrived. Fifteen people entered the same room they had used for their lecture and were greeted with their seats arranged in a circle. The "instructors" occupied two of the seats. There was silence and a little laughter. Someone then turned to one of the instructors and asked him to repeat the instructions. He smiled and noted, simply, that there was no special task agenda for them, no one was in charge, and that they could do whatever they wished to do together as a group. A bit more nervous laughter was followed by more silence. Finally, one member, Terry, decided to talk.

Terry told the group that she wanted to share a problem she was having to discover if there was any way they could help her deal with it. The problem she described involved "abandonment" and her fear of being abandoned. This was especially salient to her as she and her boyfriend of nearly two years had recently separated. She talked a bit more about abandonment and then became quiet. She had triggered a common concern and soon others had joined in the conversation. The theme continued to revolve around being abandoned, being left alone, separating from close friends, becoming independent of parents, and so on. The hour passed by quickly as nearly everyone in the group became fascinated with this theme and found themselves easily joining in the discussion.

Is there any connection between what we have just described and the idea that some events take place in groups that are unconscious, that is, that lie beyond the members' conscious awareness? We believe that there is. First, remember the situation in which the group found itself. It was their first meeting; most members were strangers to one another; they had no task or agenda; the people who were supposed to be in charge and leading the group—the two lecturers—had declined to take on this function, thus leaving the group entirely on its own. Second, recall that the theme of their conversation dealt with abandonment; being left alone and without help to deal with everything and having to grow up and become independent of parental control.

We believe that there is a definite connection between this theme and the underlying issue this group faced. We also believe that these feelings of being abandoned by those usually in control (e.g., parents, teachers) was a central element in what we will refer to as the group's *hidden agenda*; that is, the unconscious agenda this group confronted by virtue of many of its members sharing some of the same feelings, concerns, and anxieties. We likewise believe that few, if any, members were consciously aware of the connection between the theme of their conversation and the hidden agenda of their group. After all, if something is genuinely unconscious it is not therefore available for members to report as part of their awareness. Conversely, something that is unconscious is available to be discovered and thus to become part of members' conscious awareness and part of the group's stated rather than hidden agenda. Let us look a bit further at the concept, hidden agenda, and offer a few additional illustrations.

Hidden Agenda

When we talk about an unconscious process with reference to a group, just what do we mean? Without delving too deeply into the complex matter of trying to locate a group's unconscious, we will introduce the concept of the *hidden agenda* in order to sharpen our focus. Let us assume that whenever persons come together to interact, there are two levels on which that interaction takes place. That is, all group interactions involve two agendas—one conscious, often publicly stated, explicit, and open for everyone to see; the other hidden beneath the surface, implicit, closed from direct public scrutiny and awareness, but emerging nevertheless to influence whatever takes place.

Another example involves a student in a classroom who asks the teacher a question to which he already knows the answer (Yalom, 1975). On the surface, the stated agenda involves asking a question and obtaining an answer. But beneath the surface there lies another agenda. This becomes apparent when the student corrects the teacher's incorrect answer. Although all the attributes of that hidden agenda may not be known by the observer, it is a pretty good guess that it involves some effort on the part of the student to dominate or assert domination over a public authority figure. That is, the public agenda of asking a question may in this case cover a hidden agenda of attacking or challenging persons in authority.

The concept of the hidden agenda or unconscious group process is important primarily because the surface, observed behavior is not adequate to a complete understanding of the situation. Something more seems to be going on. Often, what we observe on the surface does not make much sense without an explicit concept such as that of the hidden agenda to enrich our understanding. The development of this concept of unconscious processes has emerged from many observations of many groups over a considerable period of time; it is a concept of interpretation that has been tested and typically found worthwhile.

This latter point is important. There is much resistance on the part of the beginning student and on the part of the group itself to the idea that unconscious processes may play a significant role in our behavior. Let us suppose that the teacher of the previous example not only had the suspicion about the student's "hidden agenda item" but also checked it out directly and bluntly with the student: e.g., "Are you asking me a question to which you already know the answer because you are really trying to challenge and attack me?" We would not expect the student to smile and answer, "Yes, that's it!"

Agendas are hidden from the participants as well; thus it is not reasonable to expect that a direct check will readily reveal what are often very deep lying unconscious processes. Had we pressed the point with our students concerning the idea that their hidden agenda involved their concerns over "abandonment," we would not have been likely to get direct confirmation, with all exclaiming in unison: "Yes, that's it!"

Nevertheless, concepts such as the hidden agenda can and have been tested; their overall validity as concepts necessary for understanding group process has been confirmed. Individual testing, however, cannot proceed directly. Rather, the leader or participant-observer must entertain the interpretation as a hypothesis that, if true, will be revealed in other aspects of the individual's or group's behavior.

In the example involving the question-asking student, the teacher does not ask the student if he is challenging authority, but rather asks herself what else might be true if this interpretation is valid. The teacher in this case might notice other behaviors of this same student: e.g., he comes up frequently after class to disagree about particular points that have been made; he arrives late, especially on examination days; his manner is generally antagonistic; his work is a study in a casual-to-messy style. Notice that these additional behaviors are all consistent with the preliminary interpretations; they do not prove it to be correct, but add further weight to its confirmation. And likewise, they add further weight to the teacher's use of a concept such as hidden agenda to help deepen and enrich her understanding of the particular situation she is confronting.

Basic-Assumption Group Mode

W. R. Bion, an important contributor to our understanding of group process, examines the two types of agenda in his important distinction between what he terms a *work-group* mode and a *basic-assumption* mode (Bion, 1959; also see Thelen, 1959). When a group comes together to work, it has met to do something, to accomplish a task, to cooperate in order to get a job done. Members gear themselves to reality; they focus on rational ways to complete their task; to make the decisions necessary to solve the problems they encounter; to relate in a rational way to one another. A group functioning in this way is primarily concerned with its publicly stated agenda, with the more conscious level of functioning.

But, as Bion notes, if we were to focus our attention only on the work mode in analyzing group process, we would not only miss much of what takes place, but would also fail to understand some of the issues and problems that crop up and make working together difficult. Thus, it is also necessary to attend to the kinds of *unconscious basic assumptions* that characterize group process. It was Bion's contention that there are specific, recurrent unconscious themes and issues that are basic to all groups. The unconscious emotional themes that describe the basic-assumption mode, however, involve such factors as hostility, flight or withdrawal, hope, helplessness, and dependency.

When group members glance furtively at one another while discussing the job they are doing, or when one member looks frequently at the group leader as though seeking approval, or when another member seems to reject almost automatically whatever the leader proposes, something is obviously taking place that cannot readily be understood solely in terms of the conscious task at hand. Bion suggests that concerns with leadership in particular—e.g., how to address the leader, how to handle the leader's style, what responses to make to the leader's suggestions—cannot be understood in conscious terms. Within the context of the basic-assumption mode, a group functions *as if* its members were following some shared, unconscious assumptions of why they have convened and what their purposes are. These basic assumptions are not tied into the realities at hand, nor are they designed to cope successfully with the group's tasks. Rather, they spring from deep emotional characteristics and needs within group members and tend to obstruct and divert the group from accomplishing its stated tasks.

A Critical Task

It would follow, therefore, that a critical task for a group to deal with in order to function more effectively involves understanding and working through its basic assumptions. The task or work agenda cannot be success-fully negotiated until the hidden agenda is confronted and dealt with.

The point is simple but often overlooked by more rational conceptions of group process. In this view, members' effectiveness in dealing with their tasks (i.e., the work of the group) can be thwarted by the unconscious basic assumptions of the group's hidden agenda. For example, some members may agree with the leader's directions more out of a need to be saved from feel-ing helpless and confused than because of the intrinsic merit of those sug-gestions for effectively handling the work issue that is faced. Or other members might resist good suggestions in an unconscious desire to rebel against all authority. In both cases, effective work is thwarted as members' unconscious relationships with the leader interfere with their behaving ration-ally toward their tasks.

Decisions that a group makes that primarily serve such unconscious needs will crop up again and again; thus it is easy for a group to get bogged down and become unable to move effectively unless the group confronts its hidden agenda. Similarly, the leader may get agreement that is based more on members' unconscious needs than on the merits of his or her leadership and suggestions; or the leader may meet substantial resistance that has little to do with ideas and recommendations as such. Whichever the case may be, it should be apparent that these unconscious, basic assumptions can be des-tructive to effective behavior.

Member-to-Member Transferences

While many concepts of the group's unconscious life emphasize mem-ber relationships to the leader, it is important for us to recognize that a simi-lar kind of unconscious transference can also be focused on member relationships with other members. Thus, the focus of unconscious basic assumptions is directed toward (1) the leader and (2) other members. The important unconscious themes that revolve around the leader involve mem-bers' relationships to authority, dependency, freedom, and individuality. The important themes that revolve around other members involve such issues as competition, assertiveness, intimacy, sexuality, envy, giving, sharing (Yalom, 1975). These too form part of the group's hidden agenda. They involve such factors as members' fears of competing against others and either winning or losing, or strong needs to win or lose (i.e., to fail). They may involve mem-bers' desires to be assertive or domineering. They may involve members' desires to become close and intimate with others, or fears of closeness and intimacy. They may involve members' envy of others in relation to approval of the leader, jealousies, inabilities to give and to share, and so forth.

Hidden agenda, then, provides a rich territory for exploring and understanding group process. The failure to deal with its implications and issues will inevitably cause a group to perform on a less than optimum level.

An Example

Nurse Riles has always been concerned with her femininity. She was brought up in a rather traditional way to believe that the proper role for a woman was to be relatively passive and nonassertive, especially in the presence of men. For her, being feminine is related to being nonassertive. In fact, whenever she begins to assert herself in a group she vaguely senses that she is behaving in an unfeminine manner. Consequently, she tends to altogether avoid asserting herself or she stops short just as she begins to declare her own views within the group. Nurse Riles, however, is also very frustrated and angry—especially at herself. She feels she has some good ideas to contribute. But her habitual passivity and silence makes her consent to letting others take the lead and have their ideas accepted, even when she believes that her own views may be as good and often better. Her smiling and agreeable presence is noted at group meetings; yet her underlying anger and conflict are more effective determinants of her actions. Although she may outwardly approve of the ideas that lead to a group decision, she frequently drags her feet when it is time for the final decisions to be determined. Often she is a puzzle to others in her group; they think that she is agreeing with their suggestions and yet wonder why she doesn't pitch in eagerly in following them.

In this example, we have a member's own hidden agenda, involving a link between assertiveness and femininity. This hidden agenda profoundly influences Nurse Riles's behavior within the group, and has a very detrimental effect on the whole group and it's ability to function as a unit. Decisions are made and seemingly accepted, and yet are not carried out very well. Assertiveness in this case, takes the form of an *implicit* refusal to carry out group decisions; this is covered over by what appears to be *explicit* acceptance of such decisions. That is, Nurse Riles does assert herself, but in a concealed way by her slow or grudging implementation of decisions. Clearly, a group with such members cannot hope to function well until these hidden agendas are brought to the surface so they can be dealt with; that is, until assertiveness is part of the group's explicit mode of working together.

A Summary

We have learned that all groups, no matter what their purposes may be, partake of two rather different kinds of process. The one is relatively conscious and rational and is concerned with the group's stated task agenda. This is the activity we tend to see when we observe a group in action. For example, we see the group's leader make a suggestion and members comment on it; we see decisions being made and members contributing variously to making those decisions; we see problems being discussed and solutions sought. The other process is less conscious and less rational; it reflects a set of basic assumptions under which members operate but of which they and we as casual observers tend to be unaware. More careful observation, however, may reveal that some members act as though they were angry with the leader for reasons far removed from the task at hand, or are pleased with someone else in the group—again, for reasons not immediately understandable in terms of that person's contributions to the task. Members seem to act as though guided by some basic assumptions that are less rational and more concerned with underlying emotions than those involved with their task.

We can expect hidden agendas to develop within all groups and to be focused on leadership and on other members. That is both leaders and other members serve as targets for the playing out of unconscious feelings and concerns. Typically, leaders are the focus of members' concerns with authority, freedom, and dependency; members are the focus of concerns with competition, intimacy, sharing, and such.

Work groups are always affected by basic-assumption behaviors; thus to understand and to intervene effectively in group process, we must be aware of a group's unconscious level of behavior as well as the surface manifestations of work-group activity. This is a critical point. It is not possible either to understand or effectively work with a group unless unconscious basic assumptions—the group's hidden agenda—are dealt with as they relate to conscious work and task activity.

For example, if a group's resistance to adopting a leader's suggestions is based more on unconscious than conscious reasons, no matter how hard that leader tries to rationally persuade members of the reasonableness of her suggestions, she will fail to convince. She will have invested her efforts inappropriately if she focuses on rational persuasion for issues that have an unconscious nonrational basis.

Why Hidden Agendas?

There are several reasons why all groups can be expected to develop some types of hidden agenda in addition to their publicly stated work agendas. We will briefly examine three of these reasons: unresolved feelings, learned habits of public behavior, and fears of vulnerability.

Unresolved Feelings

Most of the examples and the discussion of hidden agendas up to this point have emphasized their basis in unresolved unconscious feelings and conflicts: e.g., Nurse Riles's concern that assertiveness is not feminine. All of us arrive at our ongoing group and social settings with a variety of still unresolved issues from our past. Stock, Whitman, and Lieberman (1958) referred to these as the individual's *nuclear conflict*. They involve any number of past hurts and deprivations that remain as scars liable to be opened up again in the right situation.

Stock and her associates offer the example of a man from a large family who as a child continually tried to win the attention of his parents, to separate himself from his siblings, and to appear as someone unique and worthy of their special attention. This demand for recognition has become the adult's unresolved nuclear conflict. When this man is within a group situation, he unconsciously feels in the same competitive circumstances again—the other group members are in a sense his siblings and the leader, his parents. So he begins to strive anew for recognition and special attention; this time, however, he seeks it from the group's leader.

In other words, the group has become a setting that serves to trigger this man's unresolved conflicts; it becomes a stage upon which he plays out these unresolved underlying issues. In one way or another, we all play out such issues in our ongoing group behavior. Such nuclear issues are at the base of a group's complex constellation of hidden agendas.

Habits of Public Behavior

As we all grow up within a particular culture, we learn certain ways to publicly express our feelings and our ideas; that is, we learn certain habits of public expression. For example, some people have learned that it is not appropriate to express feelings; others have learned that feelings are something to be expressed and shared with others. Within our culture there are many, including those who enter the health professions who believe that it is not appropriate to express or share their feelings in public (Buck et al., 1974; Learmonth et al., 1959). Such people have learned to be somewhat reserved—to maintain at least a facade of calm and cool rationality.

Such behavior represents learned habits of public expression and not necessarily a manifestation of actual feelings. When individuals experience emotions but submerge them, those feelings tend to gain an indirect expression. They are thus not directly observable, but become part of the private background behavior that is influential even though "hidden." For example, Nurse Riles may have learned that she should not publicly express the anger that she feels when she fails to assert herself; but that anger does exist and is expressed indirectly in the form of reluctant, grudging compliance with decisions that are made.

Indirect expressions of feelings (or even ideas) comprise a rich source of material for a group's hidden agenda, and as such can serve to confuse and to thwart effective group communication and functioning until they are more directly confronted and dealt with.

Fears of Vulnerability

A third, related basis for the development of hidden agendas involves the fears we all have of being vulnerable. To be direct in saying what we believe or feel, for example, can open us to the possibility of attack from others. So we may choose to be indirect or to withhold in order to protect ourselves.

And yet, as we have already noted, while we do so, we become contributors to the developing hidden agenda of those groups and relationships in which we are involved.

Rational Conflicts

Not all conflicts and disagreements within groups are based on unconscious assumptions. There are many clear and definitely rational bases for disagreements; these, however, can usually be confronted directly and dealt with in a relatively reasonable manner; sensible compromises can be achieved. However, when the basis for conflict (or even for inappropriate agreement—e.g., saying "yes" to a foolish proposal) is more deeply rooted, then rational solutions are hard to achieve. Problems may recur and never be resolved; compromises may be tentative, and acceptance of leadership and of group decisions weak.

SYMBOLIZATION

An aspect of the unconscious dynamics occurring in groups that was illustrated in our earlier example of the classroom discussion of abandonment involves what can be termed the *symbolization process* (see also Mills, 1964). Nowhere are unconscious dynamics revealed more than in the symbolization of issues. A few additional examples will illustrate this.

> The group is together for its first meeting for a treatment review of Mr. R. Although several members know one another from past contacts, most are only passing acquaintances and several are new to the group. The leader, Dr. Winch, initiates the discussion about Mr. R. An intern comments on the difficulties in dealing with Mr. R. because of a language barrier. A nurse suggests that even without this barrier it would be difficult because Mr. R. speaks so softly that he is difficult to hear. Additional comments are made, all focusing on issues of communication and understanding of the patient, Mr. R.

In this example, the patient has difficulty in speaking English; he also speaks softly and people must ask him to repeat what he says. There is little doubt that one aspect of the case involves matters of communication and understanding. Yet in view of the group's interaction it appears that something more may be involved. In particular, perhaps the intensive focus on issues of communication and understanding also symbolizes or represents an underlying issue for the group. Are these doctors and nurses also introducing, via the patient's problems of communication, their own group's issues involving understanding and communication?

This appears to be a reasonable hypothesis, one that a careful analyst of group process might wish to make and to examine further. It is not surprising, of course, that persons who meet together for the first time possibly have problems in communication and understanding. This is the very type of issue that an effective group leader should look for in trying to help the group work together more effectively.

Hypothesis, Not Fact

It is important to realize that the statement that the ongoing conversation in this example symbolizes or represents an issue to the group itself is really a hunch or a hypothesis. As a hypothesis, it must both be seriously considered and tested. That is, the leader-observer must be able to formulate such hypotheses from the material of ongoing group discussion and be able to test them for their validity. But direct testing (e.g., by asking group members if they are really also talking about themselves) will not invariably confirm a correct hypothesis about symbolized, unconscious matters. In fact, there is often resistance to such interpretations.

The leader, therefore, may entertain the hypothesis but not immediately share it, deciding to wait until more material surfaces. For example, a member may eventually hint at the possibility that the members are really also talking about themselves and their own issues with one another. Or the leader may decide that it is best to intervene as though his or her interpretive hypothesis were correct. In this case the leader would assume that members are worried about their knowledge and are unsure of themselves and would thus benefit from some supportive comments from him or her. Or the leader might assume that members are having some difficulty in communicating with one another and decide to actively clarify what is being said.

Sources for Symbolization

Authority and peer relations are considered two critical areas of unconscious work within groups, and as such provide a rich source of material for frequent symbolization. We would expect groups to have discussions about problems that seem to be external to themselves (e.g., talking about Mr. R.'s communication problems) that involve issues of authority, dependency, control, freedom, and independence on the one hand, or of intimacy, friendship, acceptance, and rejection on the other. These give us a useful clue as to what issues are very likely internal to the group as well.

A student group that is about to end, for example, may talk at great length about the trouble that its patients are having with leaving the hospital after a lengthy illness. They go on and on about the patients' need for the hospital and its support, the patients' difficulties in making the break and going home again, and so forth. The hypothesis is that the group members may not only be talking about the patients' difficulties but their own difficulties in terminating their group and in leaving the friendships and support they have in the group. We might test this hypothesis by directly asking such a question as: "Is termination of our own group something that we should talk about here?" or by assuming its validity and acting upon it—e.g., "I have some feelings about our own group's ending and would like to talk about these."

A THEORY OF COLLECTIVE ANXIETY
AND ITS EFFECTS ON GROUP PROCESS

An interesting body of group and organizational research has evolved from the psychoanalytic writings of Melanie Klein (1948) as interpreted by the Tavistock Center in London. According to the theory, unconscious, primitive anxieties, which all people presumably share in common, serve as the source of many kinds of structures that emerge within groups. These anxieties also serve as barriers to organizational and group change. People cling to traditional ways of working together because those traditional ways were formed to help deal with anxiety; therefore, change is resisted because it threatens to unleash the primitive anxieties that the traditional structures had more or less successfully contained.

Two Primitive Anxieties

The theory postulates that experiences very early in all of our lives— well before we even have much more than a preliminary sense of self—create two primitive sources of anxiety. The first is centered around having too much closeness with or being engulfed by others. The second is centered around too much separation from or being estranged from others. Too much closeness versus too much separation: These are said to be primitive anxieties, originating very early in our lives and persisting in one form or another throughout.

The anxiety over too much closeness would lead us to distance ourselves from others. The anxiety over too much separation would lead us to approach others. And so, we seem caught between approaching and avoiding: too much of either triggers its opposite.

On the one hand, the anxiety over being too close leads us to adopt a kind of paranoid outlook on the world. We view others as potential sources of danger; they threaten to take us over, to engulf us. On the other hand, the anxiety over being too isolated leads us to adopt a kind of depressive attitude toward the world. We view ourselves as unworthy figures whom nobody would truly want to have nearby.

Splitting and Projective Identification

The theoretical framework we have been considering also suggests that rather than being faced with these anxieties as parts of one's self, people manage them through two unconscious psychological mechanisms. In *splitting*, the person literally splits off the bad parts of the self (e.g., I am the unworthy one, or my impulses make me the dangerous person) and then *projects* those split-off parts onto someone or something else.

A study conducted on a medical-surgical unit of a large hospital (Firman & Kaplan, 1978), for example, suggested that the job-related anxieties experienced by both physicians and nurses were managed through the dual processes of splitting and projective identification. The investigators argued that the physicians, in effect still student interns, felt very insecure about their roles and their competence in dealing with the variety of tasks they faced; the feeling of incompetence, however, was an undesirable part of themselves. The result was the splitting off of these bad elements of the self and projecting the disowned parts of the self onto the nursing staff: the nurses therefore were perceived as the ones who were insecure about their competency.

In turn, the members of the nursing staff, entirely female in this institution, had defined their own competence and assertiveness as bad qualities: these traits were not appropriate in a person who is supposedly caring and "feminine." Thus, the nurses split off their own competency and assertiveness from themselves and projected these qualities onto the physicians. They therefore saw the physicians as being highly competent and assertive—to the point of arrogance.

This example illustrates the ways in which people who work together may form relationships with their co-workers, which, deriving from splitting and projective identification, hinder the person's own development and their ability to understand and work effectively with others. In effect, relationships are not founded on the basis of reality; rather, a culture of splitting and projective identification is created that separates people from themselves and others. We will return to these concepts in the more complete illustration we provide at the end of this chapter. For now, however, we have introduced several aspects of the theory of unconscious interpersonal relationships that have some important consequences for group process. Let us now look more directly to what the theory says about group process itself.

Group Structures as a Defense Against Primitive Anxieties

The Tavistock group's argument maintains that group and organizational structures emerge as collective resolutions to our individual issues of anxiety over engulfment and estrangement; that many elements of group process likewise involve collective solutions to our individual issues of anxiety including issues that derive from the dual processes of splitting and projective identification. We have already glimpsed elements of this view in Bion's work (1959) on basic assumptions within groups to which we alluded earlier in this chapter. Let us unfold a few more details.

Several authors writing in this genre of theoretical analysis, but in particular, Bion, Slater (1966), and Thelen (1959) describe three unconscious patterns of interaction that they observed in groups, which they believe to be collective efforts to allay these anxieties: fight/flight; dependency; and pairing.

Fight/Flight

Fight/flight is considered to be a rather primitive way of dealing with anxiety, employed by human beings as well as most animal species. When anxious, we stand and fight or we run. When fight or flight becomes the prevalent manner of interaction within a group, we would suspect that the underlying issue involves the anxiety over engulfment or estrangement. In effect, too much fighting might be a group's way of avoiding getting too close. Not trusting others or feeling others are dangerous or at least potential threats to one's own integrity, one fights. The short-term success of fighting, of course, is that it does indeed separate and thus minimize the possibility of getting too close.

Some groups' collective way of coping with anxiety does not involve fighting, but rather fleeing difficult situations. Flight behavior can take several forms: no longer attending particularly troublesome meetings; leaving psychologically by daydreaming, arriving late, leaving early, being tangential, never keeping on the topic, and so forth.

Dependency

Dependency involves an admission of weakness and a submission to outside guidance. In groups, dependency is a common strategy for coping with anxiety, usually taking the form of members yielding to a leader or to a dominant individual. Rather than fighting or fleeing, members who fear either coming too close to one another or getting too far apart to function together as a group, turn to someone "superior," a "higher authority," who will protect them, keep them intact and within carefully defined limits.

It is important to note that dependency may center on a person who is the group's formal leader, on a person who emerges as dominant or protective within the group, or on anyone or anything that provides structure to the group. Recall that the primitive anxiety involves getting too close together or too far apart. Different ways of providing structure to the group help deal with either source of anxiety. Getting too close can be managed by keeping people well defined in their roles and confronting a specific task agenda that must be completed. Getting too far apart, which is a threat to the very integrity of the group, can likewise be managed by a role or task structure that keeps people together and working.

Points of structure can involve people or—in many cases—something else, such as an agenda. A group may continually refer to its past meetings or to its history as another way of providing structure. In this case, the past becomes a source of dependency, the vehicle for providing the structure that helps manage potential anxieties.

Pairing

The third form of interaction that has been posited as a collective solution to these two primitive anxieties has been called pairing. The term is simply intended to suggest how groups will often manage their problems by breaking down into smaller subgroups, with the pair being the smallest subgroup prior to total group dissolution. As long as individuals can work together in smaller subgroups, they may feel themselves protected from the more formidable tensions resulting from having to interact within a larger group.

A HEALTH-CARE ILLUSTRATION

So that the abstractions that are an inevitable part of any theoretical statement will not interfere with understanding how this theory operates in practice, we have chosen an example that emerged some years ago as part of the Tavistock Center's efforts to apply its theoretical scheme to an actual organizational problem. The example is based on the research reported by Isabel Menzies (1960) in her study of the nursing service of a general teaching hospital in London.

The teaching hospital in which the research was conducted contained 500 beds, and additionally included three smaller specialist hospitals and an adjoining convalescent home. There were about 700 nursing personnel, 150 of whom were fully trained senior staff, the remainder of whom were nurses in training. The senior nursing staff were primarily involved in administrative activities and teaching, while the students were involved in direct patient care. The nursing service emphasized patient care, making the training function secondary. This feature produced a continuing series of crises: senior staff were eager to provide more training in order to improve the skills of the student nurses, while the institutional demand was centered around providing patient care with a lesser concern for training.

Menzies was called in as a consultant to the nursing service when senior nursing staff became concerned that the service was heading towards a complete breakdown: the demands for patient care were beginning to overwhelm the possibilities for providing quality training to the student nurses. Menzies began her work at the hospital by conducting intensive interviews with both individuals and small groups of nurses, medical, and nonprofessional staff. She also observed the hospital.

Both interviews and observation exposed high levels of tension and anxiety among the nurses, including such signs of job stress as: high rates of withdrawal from their duties; the voluntarily departure of approximately one-third of the students from the training program; senior staff members frequently changing their jobs or seeking further training so that they, too, could get out of this situation; high rates of illness in the nursing service.

In reflecting on this disabling degree of stress within the nursing service, Menzies called upon the theoretical framework we have been considering in this chapter, particularly the Kleinian notions of primitive anxieties, splitting, and the role of organizational structures in containing those anxieties. Menzies suggested that the primary task of patient care itself arouses substantial primitive anxieties among the caregivers (i.e., the nurses in training). Being in constant contact with people who are ill or dying is stressful in itself. Seeing the patients' dependency and constant need for attention arouses a mixture of feelings among the caregivers including compassion and pity on the one hand, and resentment and envy on the other. The struggling nurses, in fact, envied some of the special care and attention lavished on the patients that they wished they too could sometimes receive.

Furthermore, seeing the patients and their families in so needy a condition, sensing their own inability to alleviate all the pain they had to deal with on a daily basis and being vaguely reminded of their own early fantasies about doing harm to others they really cared about, the student nurses were frequently anxious. In Menzies analysis, the patients were like an *alloy*, a combination of the real and the imagined patient derived from the nurses' own primitive anxieties. All of this combined to further deepen the stress of their job.

Menzies called upon the next element in the theoretical framework she was using to diagnose the problems she encountered. She reasoned that the structure of the nursing service was somehow helping defend against these anxieties she had identified.

> A social defense system develops over time as the result of collusive interaction and agreement, often unconscious, between members of the organization as to what form it shall take. The socially structured defense mechanisms then tend to become an aspect of external reality with which old and new members of the institution must come to terms (p. 101).

In effect, Menzies was suggesting that the nursing service at this teaching hospital was set up as a social defense against primitive anxieties; that "the nursing service makes use of other people, notably patients and doctors, in operating socially structured mechanisms of defense" (p. 101).

Her next task was to take another look at some of the activities that occurred within the nursing service, now framed within this theoretical perspective: that is, to see how the nurses' everyday activities might be understood as devices to help defend against primitive anxieties. A sampling of some of Menzies's analyses will prove helpful.

Menzies argued that the process of *depersonalization* is one device that helped the nursing staff deal with anxiety. This involved relating to fragmented patients rather than whole individuals: dealing, for example, with the gallbladder in room #101, not Mrs. Smith. This also involved detaching oneself from pain and suffering by denying feelings that, if not denied, might overwhelm.

Detachment also took on another form as nurses defined the "good nurse" as one who does not mind moving about from task to task, from patient to patient, never pausing long enough to get involved with any one patient. Therefore, to be a "good nurse," the individual had to keep in motion to the extent that one never became involved with any one patient and thereby risk feeling something about this person.

Menzies also reasoned that in defining her job as a technical matter, the nurse's anxiety could be contained. The technical focus helps reduce the anxiety that stems from exercising one's discretion in being responsible for the patient's fate.

A related feature of the situation involved what Menzies termed the *culture of splitting*. We already saw this culture functioning in the research reported by Firman and Kaplan. The nursing task places the individual in a difficult situation. On the one hand, the nurse does bear a significant burden of responsibility for the care of her patients. On the other hand, especially for someone in the process of training, there is always the temptation to give up this burden, to be less responsible, to give in to impulses, and even to lose the detachment that is part of her work with patients. The structure of the hospital had built in an externalization of these conflicting feelings and so helped reduce the likelihood that the conflict would be experienced internally.

Some roles within the hospital were defined as "responsible," while others, "nonresponsible." "Nurses habitually complain that other nurses are irresponsible, behave carelessly and impulsively, and in consequence must be ceaselessly supervised and disciplined" (p. 105). What occurs is a dichotomy both within the objective hospital situation and within the nurse herself. This involves viewing the senior staff as responsible and competent and the student nurses as irresponsible and noncompetent. Insofar as each student nurse experienced the culture in this manner, she tended to define bad nurses as the junior staff, while seeing her superiors as models of the good nurse.

> Each nurse tends to split off aspects of herself from her conscious personality and to project them onto other nurses. Her irresponsible impulses, which she fears she cannot control, are attributed to her juniors. Her painfully severe attitude to these impulses and burdensome sense of responsibility are attributed to her seniors (p. 105).

The outcome of this culture of splitting is that the nurses treat their juniors very harshly and expect to be treated harshly by the senior staff. None of this is conducive to positive working relationships and indeed contributes significantly to the high levels of tension and stress that Menzies observed in this hospital's nursing service.

Another consequence of the preceding situation (e.g., the culture of splitting plus the other features we have introduced), is that any change in procedure is difficult, if not impossible, to make, largely because the current structures serve as defenses against the anxieties that would be unleashed were new structures or procedures instituted.

Menzies reports several attempts, for example, to give clerical staff some administrative tasks that the already overburdened senior staff did not really need to continue performing. When junior staff greeted this change with anger and upset, the senior staff agreed to continue with things as usual. In Menzies's view, the resistance of the junior staff to this change involved its deep (and unconscious) projection of high levels of competence onto the senior staff, and its fears about the chaos they assumed would occur if the senior staff did not continue to make even clerical decisions. The example also illustrates the collusive alliance between junior and senior staff as the latter accepted its burdensome role in response to what it sensed to be the anguish of the junior staff.

Before we leave this example and the role of unconscious processes in groups, we need to note, along with Menzies, one further feature of the case she analyzed. On the one hand, we speak of the structures of this organization serving as defenses against anxiety; we suggest that resistance to change is a function of peoples' clinging to old structures that help contain their anxieties. On the other hand, we simultaneously refer to this organization as being so beset with anxiety and tension that it is near the breaking point. How can this be? That is, how can structures contain anxiety and yet obviously not do so successfully?

For the most part, the institutional structures Menzies has described merely cover anxiety rather than help individuals master it. Thus not only does the anxiety disperse, causing additional tension within the system, but, in never being addressed directly, is also never brought under conscious control. Furthermore, as we have seen, the resistance to any change within the organization makes it difficult to introduce new approaches that might help people master the anxiety. Thus, arrangements are perpetuated that are, in the long run, dysfunctional for effective practice.

CONCLUSION

This chapter has introduced the student to the idea that some of the processes that take place within groups occur at a level below direct awareness, that these unconscious processes within groups can play an important role in shaping the groups' effectiveness in dealing with its professional tasks (e.g., patient care), and in serving the many other functions a group plays for its members and the organization within which it is located. We devoted considerable space to the case illustration provided by Menzies in order to demonstrate how one theory about these unconscious processes has been employed to diagnose a particularly troublesome situation in the nursing service of a large training hospital.

The analysis suggests that the consultant, Menzies in this case, has a difficult task ahead in helping to reorient the nursing service by some rather lengthy and complex interventions that demand a level of knowledge and skill usually well beyond the introductory student's capabilities. We are not recommending that beginning students, armed only with this brief introduction to the world of unconscious dynamics within groups, boldly step forth to restructure their own groups' unconscious dynamics. We hope rather, that we have sensitized students to another way of understanding some of what takes place in groups; and perhaps even motivated a few to study further so that the special expertise required to deal with unconscious processes can eventually become part of their repertoire of skills.

9

Intergroup Relations

As we noted in Chapter 2, one result of the recent health-care revolution in the United States has been its impact on intergroup relations. When professionals work in a corporate environment, they quickly become sensitive to the importance of their own and of others' group memberships as central elements in their professional lives and practices. But, it is not only the health-care revolution that has increased the relevance of intergroup relations to our lives. Several additional factors need to be noted, if only briefly.

Our world has grown significantly smaller as the technologies of transportation and communication have brought us into contact with peoples and places once beyond our reach. We have become increasingly aware of many differences between ourselves and others and have begun to learn about the important role that our memberships in particular groups and cultures play in our lives.

Never before in human history have we seen so clearly the division of the world into "haves" and "have-nots"—majority groups and nations with power and plenty as opposed to minority groups and nations with few opportunities or hope. In fact, intergroup relations and conflicts between groups rather than individuals have become a salient feature of our everyday world.

Finally, the 1960s in the United States witnessed the emergence of a variety of political and social movements seeking to provide certain groups with rights and benefits that had long been denied to them: the struggle for civil rights for African-Americans and for other people of color; the battle for women's rights; the continuing conflicts over gay and lesbian rights; the efforts to bring the handicapped into the mainstream of American life. These and other struggles have given us a higher awareness of the important role that our group memberships play in our daily lives and in the lives of those that live and work with us.

Those entering the 1990s with an interest in group process must therefore come to terms with the growing importance of intergroup relations as a central element of their knowledge.

Recall the lesson from Chapter 3, in which we suggested that there are two perspectives one can adopt when examining group process: focusing on individual level processes and focusing on group level processes. It is clear that when our concern lies with intergroup relations, our emphasis must be directed primarily toward group level processes, specifically the relations among and between individuals who are defined by their group memberships. Whenever we deal with intergroup relations, therefore, we are concerned with persons whose group memberships are features integral to our understanding. Let us illustrate with an example borrowed and somewhat modified from one of the textbooks in this area (Taylor and Moghaddam, 1987).

A young couple is having a romantic dinner at a local restaurant. Their conversation wends its way through various topics, moving rather easily from the weather and the day's work toward things a bit more personal and intimate. At this moment, they are relating to each other primarily on a purely individual level. But then—seemingly out of the blue—the young man makes a remark about one of the patrons seated at a nearby table that his date perceives as sexist. Suddenly, the couple's relationship undergoes a change. The young woman, now experiencing herself as a feminist and her date as a sexist, begins to relate to him less as an intimate than as a member of a particular group. He, in turn, becomes somewhat defensive at these changes in the way she is relating to him, and so begins to deal with her as a member of a feminist subculture. The example illustrates how a relationship transforms quite suddenly, from one of individuals relating to one another as individuals into one of persons relating to one another in terms of their group memberships.

Many relationships, of course, begin and end as intergroup, never having been transformed as in the previous example. Consider the number of situations in our everyday lives, both privately and professionally, in which our group memberships stand out as beacons defining us. We may wear uniforms or other symbols that designate our memberships; we may use titles in addition to our name in order to provide a membership category; or early in a conversation with someone who does not know us, we may announce our occupation, thus placing ourselves within a system of memberships. In these and many other ways, some of which are not readily within our control—e.g., our gender, our skin color, our native accent—we become members of groups relating to others and being related to by others in terms of our group categories.

GROUP IDENTIFICATION AND INTERGROUP RELATIONS

At this point, many may be wondering what difference group membership identification makes? Does it really matter to people once my group category or theirs is identified? Surely, we will continue to relate to one another as unique individuals, not as anonymous members of a category! In order to study the consequences of intergroup identification, a group of investigators, led in great measure by Tajfel and his colleagues (Tajfel, 1978a; 1978b;

Billig, 1976) provide us some helpful answers.

One of the most striking and consistent research findings is an inter-group biasing effect. Once individuals categorize themselves and others on the basis of group memberships, there is a strong tendency both to differen-tiate ingroup from outgroup and to make biased judgments in favor of the ingroup. In other words, the tendency is to see members of the ingroup in a positive light when compared to persons identified as members of the out-group. The effect tends to be so pronounced that even a seemingly trivial basis for membership (e.g., sharing the same aesthetic judgments or similar judgments on an experimental estimation task) will bring out the favorable ingroup biasing effect.

The biasing itself further influences a broad range of judgments that persons make about "their own kind" in contrast with "others." Several inves-tigations have revealed the tendency for persons to judge the "same" act when performed by an ingroup member as being reasonable and proper and as improper or unreasonable when performed by an outgroup member (Dun-can, 1976; Taylor & Jaggi, 1974). It is clear that an action becomes assimilated to the social group performing that action.

An illustration of this tendency to frame the same action differently as a function of the group membership of the persons involved can be found in Duncan's research (1976). It is typical of most of the work that reveals this same effect. Duncan asked a sample of white college students to look at a videotape of an argument between two men, one of whom was white, the other of whom was black. Toward the end of the argument, one of the men shoved the other man. In half of the video tapes, the shoving was done by the black man; in the other half of the tapes, it was done by the white man. The subjects were asked to rate the degree of violence involved in this situa-tion. Of those subjects who saw a videotape in which the white man shoved the black man, 17 percent called the act violent. Of those who saw the ver-sion in which the black man shoved the white, 75 percent called the act vio-lent. Remember that all subjects were white. This research illustrates the tendency people have to rate a behavior performed by an ingroup member more favorably (i.e., less violent in this case) than the same behavior performed by an outgroup member. At this point, several conclusions seem warranted.

First, the tendency to organize our social world into ingroups and out-groups by categorizing self and others on the basis of group memberships, appears to be a pervasive quality of most human relationships.

Second, once we have divided the world into these broad categories, we tend to rate our ingroup more favorably than we do the outgroup.

Third, we tend to frame the same behaviors differently as a function of the membership of the person doing the action. An action performed by an ingroup member is viewed in a more approving light than the same action performed by an outgroup member.

Fourth, and finally, given the preceding, it should be apparent that the stereotypes we form about persons as a function of their group member-ships will be resistant to change merely by interacting with these persons. If we reframe the behavior of others to fit the stereotype we have of their group, we are unlikely to undo the stereotype's hold on us. If our stereotype of blacks is that they are more violent than whites, then, as Duncan's research suggests, we use this stereotype to frame the behavior of whites and blacks differently, and so perpetuate the effect of that stereotype on our under-standing (also see Pettigrew, 1979).

It should also be apparent that if the trivial bases for establishing group membership that are used in some of the laboratory research can call forth such strong biasing effects, then surely the kinds of categorization that we encounter in our everyday lives must be even more potent. Categorization and its biasing effects are the very conditions that can produce conflicts between groups. One way that people may increase the favorableness of their ingroup is by denigrating the outgroup. Let us look at another research example from social psychology.

GROUPS IN HARMONY AND TENSION

In what has become a classic study, two social psychologists, Carolyn and Muzafer Sherif (1953; M. Sherif, 1966), created a real life situation in which intergroup dynamics played a central part. The Sherifs ran a summer camp for young boys and were therefore able to create various conditions of living, working, and playing at the camp that provided a natural research site for their investigations. After the campers had been together for a period of time and had formed spontaneous friendship groups among themselves, Sherif divided them into two groups. The division was such that the majority of the original, spontaneous friendship groups were separated into different cabins.

After the separation, boys who had previously chosen their friends from anywhere in the camp, restricted their friendship choices to members of their ingroup. Reflect for a moment on this finding. When left on their own, without any particular basis for being divided into ingroups versus outgroups, the boys chose their friends spontaneously. Once an ingroup-outgroup distinc-tion had been created, however, friendship choices shifted perceptibly: former friends were dropped; ingroup choices predominated.

In another phase of this same research project, Sherif created a series of tasks that required the boys to work together in teams: performing, for example, tasks involving cooking, building, and so forth. After a brief time, each team developed its own ingroup identity, with special names for its mem-bers, symbols depicting the group and ways of working together. Once it became known to the boys that there were several teams, the familiar ingroup versus outgroup biasing effects emerged. Competition and intense rivalry developed between the teams; loyalty to one's own team and denigration of the opposing team also emerged in a predictable manner. Ingroup task successes were overvalued while outgroup successes were undervalued.

As the intensity of the conflict between the teams grew (threatening to split the camp apart) the Sherifs devised a plan to create harmony out of this conflict. Their idea was simple, and possible to interpret on the basis of the theoretical ideas with which we have been dealing. If ingroups and outgroups make biased judgments of their members, then if a single ingroup could be created, the conflict between groups might vanish. The Sherifs established a superordinate goal that demanded that all the campers work together in order to reach it. By creating a series of camp crises that required everyone to work together on behalf of the superordinate goal of resolving the crisis (e.g., trouble with the entire camps water supply), the Sherifs demonstrated how harmony could be restored out of what had once been an excessively tense, high-conflict situation. In effect, the superordinate goals had created one large ingroup, thus undermining the ingroup versus outgroup biasing effects that had previously wracked the camp with conflict.

INTERGROUP CONFLICTS OF INTEREST

In many instances in our lives and professional practice, the ingroup-outgroup distinction is based on a real conflict of interest between our group and another. When we refer to an interest that a group of people might have, we do not mean anything more mysterious than the fact that some outcomes would prove more beneficial to the group than others. It would be in the interest of the group, therefore, to strive for those outcomes that are to their benefit. When we speak of a conflict of interest between two groups, we then mean that one group's preferred outcomes may be at odds with another's. In other words, in order for Group A to get what it wants, Group B may not get all that it too wants.

If all of life were a win-lose affair, in which one group's getting its preferred outcomes deprived another of its preferred outcomes, then we would truly live in a state of anarchy, with no method of meaningful cooperation. In reality, however, the typical situation involves a nonzero-sum relationship: one group's interests cannot be entirely satisfied without simultaneously satisfying some of another group's interests and vice versa. In effect, the two groups need to work together in some manner if either is to achieve the outcomes it wishes.

Every hospital, for example, requires cooperation between managerial and professional staff in order for the hospital to function. Although there may be a conflict of interest between the business managers' desire to make unlimited profits for the corporation and the professional staff's concern with providing good quality patient care, it is obvious that neither party can realize its interests without working cooperatively with the other. The business managers cannot simply ignore professional advice as they seek to maximize their profits. The professional staff, in turn, cannot accomplish quality health care that is entirely oblivious to costs and profit margins. It needs the hospital and its profit-making system in order to provide the best care possible to its patients. In this case, neither group can realize its interests without reaching an agreement with the other. Indeed, if either group were to pursue its own interests without due regard for the interests of the other, the entire system would soon fall apart.

To this point, we have introduced two main ideas. First, we noted that groups have interests that may be in conflict with the interests of other groups. We also noted, though, that unless each group can work with the other group, no one's interests are likely to be met. The ingroup biasing effect we considered earlier in this chapter may hinder the very cooperation between groups that is needed if either group is to achieve its own interests.

We have, until this point, ignored several important elements that are involved when a group seeks to achieve its own interests. The simple notion of group interest conceals points that we must examine. Although a group may have interests, this does not necessarily mean that all of its members will recognize those interests, that the group will be sufficiently well organized or will be powerful enough to advocate on behalf of its own interests.

Awareness

Acting in terms of even a personal interest let alone a group interest is not possible without an awareness of that interest. On the individual level, it is not unusual to find some people acting in ways contrary to their own interests. Certain health habits, such as smoking, reflect the fact that despite an awareness of the harmful effect of such habits, this knowledge may not be sufficient in and of itself to change an individual's behavior.

When we are dealing with groups, the issue of awareness becomes a trifle more clouded. Who, in a group, must have this awareness of the group interest? Everyone? The leader? A ruling clique? Unfortunately, there are no simple answers. Clearly, however, if no member of the group is aware of what would be to the best interest of the group, then action on behalf of serving that interest is unlikely. On the other hand, if only the group leader is aware, her awareness will not invariably translate into group action unless she can help the members achieve a comparable awareness.

Organization

Awareness of an interest, whether individual or group, might in itself prove more frustrating than empowering, unless there is an organized capability to advance that interest. While individuals may be aware of what is best for them, they may be unable to put this awareness into action. Groups are not that different. Unless people who become aware that they share a common fate with their fellows can become sufficiently organized to translate that awareness into a program of action, little is likely to follow. In health care, for example, most consumers are well aware of the skyrocketing costs and even have become suspicious of the quality of the care they are receiving; yet, they remain more a collection of frustrated individuals who share a common fate than an organized collective formed into a consumer movement seeking to induce change in the health-care system.

Power

Awareness and organization are important elements in galvanizing a group to action on behalf of realizing its interests, but without the requisite power such action might be a quixotic flailing at windmills. Power appears in a variety of forms. Its absence in any form is conducive to resignation to one's fate rather than action designed to meet collective needs. Likewise, power is an important element in the process of coordination between two groups. If one group has the power to get what it wants, disregarding another's interests entirely, there is little need for anything more than a zero-sum, win-lose outlook. We return again to these ideas in chapter 10.

When we think of power, we often take a negative view: X has power over Y, fundamentally, because X can do grave harm to Y. While this kind of ability to punish another is indeed an important source of power, there are other sources that may be equally potent and even more effective in the long run. A group may have great power to punish and therefore never strike a deal with those in weaker positions. It may win in the short run only to provoke a revolution in the long run. The powerful therefore lose everything for their one brief moment in the sun. Let us now examine several bases of power that are not so firmly rooted in the ability to punish.

If I can reward you for your compliance with my requests, then I have power over you. If you happen to like me or possibly even identify with me, then I can use that as a basis of power over you. My expertise in a given area gives me still another source of power over you (see French & Raven, 1959, for a summary of these several bases of power). There is yet another kind of power that appears routinely but does not involve threats, rewards, liking, or expertise. This is the power to set the terms of an agenda or define the terms by which any given aspect of reality is understood.

Control over the agenda of a meeting, for example, is a vital source of power that some people have over others. The agenda can limit what is legitimate to talk about, the order in which items are addressed and even the amount of time available to deal with any given item. If an item that is especially relevant to one groups' interests is left off the agenda, then, by that deletion, its interests will not be handled at this particular meeting.

A form of power that relates to the preceding is based on being able to set the terms by which reality gets defined. Consider, for example, the power that one group has in defining the abortion issue by the term, pro-life. Reflect on how the opposing group, known as being in favor of the rights of individual women to have choice in this matter, has sought to regain the upper hand of public opinion by defining its view as being, pro-choice. Two very different ways to define reality: life versus choice. Each group seeks to use these terms in its efforts to win over converts to its way of thinking.

Intergroup relations are a plentiful source of further examples of this kind of reality-framing power, in which the powerful group attempts to define the terms by which the demands of the less powerful are to be understood. It comes as no surprise to learn that the group in Nation Y, whose side we support, has been labeled by our government as freedom fighters, while Nation Y's own government refers to them as terrorists. Each term calls forth a very different framing of reality and invites a very different kind of treatment: Provide aid for the freedom fighters; destroy the terrorists.

Those in charge of organizations may try to define terms so that the interests of the less powerful are said to be selfish rather than their own, which are deemed altruistic. Or, they may suggest that the motivations of the less powerful are biased and distorted, while their own interests are motivated only by their humanitarian concerns. In these and other ways, power gets wielded by virtue of those holding that power being able to control how reality is framed.

Ask any woman who has tried to be heard in certain groups what it feels like to have the men in charge of the group call her "pushy" or "aggressive." Should she want to advocate strongly on behalf of her own group's needs, she finds herself referred to as excessively narrow and egocentric. If she wants to hear all sides before making up her mind, she finds herself described as indecisive and insecure. When she wants to have more time to herself and her family, she is described as "unprofessional, "immature," or possibly "the way women are." In these and other ways, the very terms of the debate are defined by those in more powerful positions. Once people accept the powerful group's framing of the situation, they become caught in a trap from which escape is highly difficult.

Power involves many different processes. Without power, however, a group's interests are not likely to be met, even if the group has member awareness of common interests and has become organized to pursue those interests.

SOCIAL COMPARISON AND RELATIVE DEPRIVATION

We previously introduced the idea that once group memberships become relevant, people behave towards one another in terms of those memberships, typically, by overly valuing their ingroup and derogating the outgroup. As we have just noted, however, people may also be driven to action on the basis of ingroup-outgroup comparisons that reveal their group to be at some kind of disadvantage. In other words, rather than experiencing the ingroup to be "the best," the observation is made that the ingroup is relatively disadvantaged when compared to the outgroup. Early research carried out during and after World War II provided an important demonstration of what has come to be known as *relative deprivation* (Stouffer, et al., 1949a: 1949b)

Two findings from Stouffer's research demonstrated this phenomenon of intergroup comparison. Each finding suggests that regardless of the so-called "objective reality" of their circumstances, people tend to make comparisons of their own situation vis-à-vis the situation of a relevant comparison group, seeing themselves to be relatively deprived (i.e., relatively disadvantaged). (1) Married men more often questioned the legitimacy of their induction into the service than single men. (2) Men in the Air Force—where actual chances for promotion were high as compared with men in the Military Police, whose promotional chances were extremely low—felt that their own chances for promotion were very low.

A married soldier, comparing himself to his married civilian friends, felt that his induction into the army was a great sacrifice. He felt deprived when he compared his fate with theirs. The second example illustrates another facet of the relative deprivation effect: People who expect to be promoted, but are not, feel worse off than people who do not expect to be promoted, and are not.

The phenomenon of relative deprivation teaches us that we are always engaged in a process of social comparison, judging the value of our own standing vis-à-vis the standing of comparison groups. For the most part, the examples emphasize comparisons that an individual makes of his or her own standing. In 1966, Runciman added to this picture by distinguishing between what he termed *egoistical* deprivation and *fraternal* deprivation. The former is well illustrated by the examples we cited from Stouffer's work. Egoistical deprivation involves the individual's own sense of frustration over comparisons that lead him or her to feel relatively deprived.

Fraternal deprivation occurs when a person's group appears disadvantaged when compared to other groups in society. Taylor and Moghaddam (1987) offer a simple example that joins both concepts of relative deprivation. A woman might feel herself to be relatively deprived when comparing her earnings at work with others where she works: egoistical deprivation. However, she might also feel that women as a group are relatively deprived when their wages are compared with men doing the same kinds of work in society: fraternal deprivation.

The opportunities for experiencing both of these kinds of intergroup deprivations within organizational settings in which health professionals work are legion. Nurses individually can compare their employment situations, including both pay and working conditions, with other health professionals. In terms of egoistic deprivation, some individual nurses may feel themselves to be worse off in Hospital A when compared to nurses they know who are working in Hospital B. Or, some may feel that the conditions on their floor are worse than the conditions on another floor. With respect to fraternal deprivation (a possibly poor choice of terms, given its male-centered orientation), nurses as a group may not feel that they are paid what they properly deserve when comparing themselves to other occupations in society or, for that matter, with other health-care providers.

Patients may also be involved in these kinds of social comparisons. One patient may feel that he would get better care were he in another hospital or he may feel that another patient is getting more attention than he is. Given the dependency that occurs within most medical settings, it is also possible that a kind of sibling rivalry reminiscent of the family will emerge among patients, producing many kinds of invidious comparisons. Although these illustrate egoistic comparisons, as noted earlier in this chapter, it is always possible for patients to organize and seek redress for their grievances. They might compare their fate as consumers with other kinds of consumers and believe themselves to be relatively disadvantaged in the health-care system.

SUMMARY AND CONCLUSIONS

Once we remove the cultural blinders that dispose us to focus on the individual, we begin to see a bit more clearly both group processes and, as in this chapter, intergroup processes. The emphasis on intergroup relations is concerned with what happens once we define ourselves and others in terms of our group memberships, no longer relating to one another simply as specific individuals—Jane or Bill—but as representatives of specific groups, i.e., single women or black men. As our professional lives become increasingly fragmented into a variety of group memberships, and as each of those memberships comes increasingly to define a specific interest we share with others who are similarly situated, the need to understand intergroup dynamics becomes even greater than previously considered.

In this chapter, we have seen the significant tendency to divide the world into ingroups and outgroups and, once having made that division, to inflate the merits of our ingroup and to deflate the qualities of the outgroup. Many social phenomena involving stereotyping and intergroup conflicts between majorities and minorities come from this tendency to categorize ourselves and others in terms of group memberships. As we have seen, this same process of social categorization can also produce social movements designed to improve the lot of the disadvantaged. In other words, social change can also flow from the same dynamics that produce ingroup-outgroup comparisons in the first place.

Given the increasingly differentiated organizational environments within which health professionals work and the growing sensitivity to the social categories that locate persons—male, female, gay, lesbian, straight, white, black, asian, hispanic, Christian Moslem, Jew, etc.—understanding the ways in which intergroup relations operate will become increasingly relevant to our daily work. One of the primary issues, of course, involves working through some of these categorizations in order to develop ways of working together. This leads us to the topic of *negotiation,* we will consider next in Chapter 10.

IV

Dealing with Practical Issues in Group Process

The four chapters included in this final section attempt to answer some of the nagging questions we all have about groups: What should we do? How do we intervene? How do we deal with this or that issue? Unfortunately, those who are seeking a recipe book that outlines how to deal with every problem that ever has or ever will arise in groups, and provides a sure-fire formula for handling each problem, will find this section a disappointment. People—individually or collectively—pose a never-ending challenge that is ever-moving in new directions. The moment we believe we finally understand, people—cognizant of that understanding—move yet one step beyond. This universal feature renders obsolete any formula-directed recipe book even before it has been printed. What we do provide in this unit, however, are some important guidelines for understanding and intervention. Chapter 10 examines negotiation, presenting both the central issues that are involved and suggesting some helpful ways to improve the outcomes of any negotiation process.

Chapter 11 is designed to improve our abilities to observe behavior in groups and suggests ways to increase our diagnostic skills, while Chapter 12 examines the complexities involved in group leadership and recommends some techniques for improving one's own leadership skills. Finally, Chapter 13 provides a highly realistic series of key questions and answers regarding specific types of problems one is likely to encounter in groups.

10

Negotiation

*F*ew things are more significant to nearly every aspect of our modern world than negotiation: the collective search for a resolution to a disagreement between individuals or groups. Negotiation occurs everyday in our personal and our professional lives. "What should we do tonight?" This simple question posed to one friend by another initiates a process of negotiation as the two parties seek to agree on their evening's plans. In the area of group process—particularly intergroup relations—negotiation stands as a matter of prime importance.

In Chapter 2 we introduced a situation needing negotiation: a disagreement between physicians, who wanted the nursing staff to take each patient's vital signs every four hours, and the nursing staff, who felt this schedule was not only unnecessary for the majority of patients, but would soon interrupt their other activities. Every hospital policy and every change in hospital policy required the approval of a committee composed entirely of physicians. This brought all aspects of nursing practice under the governance of the physicians. Therefore, the only way for the nursing staff to change the policy involving the taking of vital signs, would be to negotiate that change with the physicians and bring a joint, nurse-physician recommendation for a new policy to the governing committee of physicians.

In this hospital, the governing committee of physicians was under the rule of an administrative committee composed entirely of corporate executives in charge of this and other hospitals owned by the national corporation. Negotiation between the professional medical staff and management was thereby also a central feature of the everyday functioning of this hospital's organization.

SOME CHARACTERISTICS OF A
NEGOTIATION SITUATION

As the preceding examples illustrate, a situation involves negotiation whenever there is a difference between two parties who must work out the terms for their continuing relationship. The physicians and nurses must continue to work together and must therefore negotiate a way to deal with the differences that currently divide them. Business management and physicians must continue to work together and so must negotiate a means to deal with whatever differences divide them. Obviously, when there are no differences between the parties or where they have no need to continue working or living together, there is little or no need for negotiation.

In human affairs, differences between two individuals or two groups can occur for any number of reasons. We may prefer different things than others do; if we wish to continue working together, we must find some manner of minimizing the conflicts that these different preferences create. For example, one partner wants to vacation in the mountains while the other would prefer the seashore. Clearly, unless they are to become immobilized by these differences, the couple must work out some kind of compromise, in which they each give a little in order to continue to function together.

We may also differ from others in our beliefs or opinions. Once again, if these differences hinder our ability to work effectively together, then we must enter into some kind of negotiation with them. Clearly, not every difference in attitudes, beliefs, or opinions requires negotiation.

If I believe that a freemarket economy is the only way to run the country and you believe that firm governmental regulation is required, this difference may or may not be cause for you and me to negotiate some resolution. If we are both members of a committee whose task has very little to do with those beliefs, then it is likely we can function effectively together without ever having to have our negotiations influenced by those issues. However, if you and I are on a committee establishing hospital economic policy or if I represent top corporate management and you are a member of a Congressional Committee reviewing national health-care policy, then these differences in attitude may well affect our negotiations.

Negotiation Issues

A difference in interests between individuals or groups (recall the discussion in Chapter 9) will be the primary reason that negotiation is likely to be required. The mountain vs. seashore example could be seen as illustrative of this point for individuals. Because of their different preferences, the two parties have interests that would lead to different outcomes. Likewise, the physicians and nurses have different sets of interests involved in the taking of vital signs. Both groups cannot achieve the outcome they believe meets their groups' interests. Some negotiation is therefore required.

Although a complete list of interests that might divide people is not possible to produce, we can outline four central themes around which negotiation is very likely to occur.

Money and Resources

People want to receive their fair share of whatever money or other resources is properly due to them. Many conflicts between individuals and groups arise over how much each party receives, how it was decided to divide the resources in that manner, and whether or not the allocation is fair.

Revolutions have been triggered by the "have-nots" finally seeking to overthrow "the haves," in order to provide a more equitable allocation of a nation's resources. Labor strikes have likewise been driven by an effort to improve the workers' pay and working conditions. Justice—whether involving the fairness by which resources have been distributed (Cohen, 1987) or the procedures by which resources have been allocated (Tylor, 1987)—is a primary source of disagreement and conflict between individuals, groups and nations, and a clear area for important negotiations.

In the area of health care, conflicts and negotiations over resource allocation are central in the lives of providers, corporate management, and consumers. Access to quality services, the cost of those services, decision-making, and allocation of the monies charged for those services, are all issues vital to national health-care policy, involving most of us as citizens and as professionals. The entire September issue of *The Journal of Justice Research* (Lichtman & Wolfe, 1987) is devoted to a discussion of these issues and provides a helpful source of information for the interested student.

Power and Control

Having a voice in decisions and being in charge of our own lives are issues central to most of our lives today and an important source of disagreement, conflict, and negotiation. Underlying many disagreements, for example, is the issue of control: Who decides? Who is really in charge around here? Participation in decision-making is a theme central to most theories of group and organizational leadership and continues to be a source of many of the issues that divide people and compel negotiation (e.g., see our discussion in Chapter 12).

Security

Few people enjoy living their lives on the edge, never quite knowing what is next in store for them, where their next meal will come from, where they will be sleeping that night, and so forth. We want to be secure in our employment and in our overall living conditions. Disagreements and conflicts arise, making negotiation important, whenever we feel that our security is threatened.

We are well aware of the importance of security in international relations, in which one nation, sensing that its integrity is threatened by the activities of an adjoining nation, may even go to war to maintain the security of its borders or supply lines. A similar concern with maintaining security occurs between individuals and between groups. For example, when the employment status of nurses in one unit is threatened by the cost-conscious management decision to employ a greater number of less well-trained and less costly nursing assistants, a situation ripe for negotiation is created. We will return to this example later in this chapter.

Respect

Differing from money, which is tangible and can actually be gathered and held, respect is, nevertheless, a vital component in our lives and a never-ending source of conflict between individuals and between groups. Concerns over receiving proper respect thereby provides still another important source of issues around which negotiation is likely to take place.

Most people want to be accorded respect and be treated decently and honorably simply because they are human beings. Just being a person is often felt to be sufficient warrant to not be treated in a shabby manner by one's fellow workers or one's supervisors or, in fact, by anyone in the work environment. The workplace is a setting in which lack of respect is often an issue that divides people, leading to hurt feelings and a general climate of distrust and alienation. An important theme in intergroup relations revolves around the failure of one party to accord respect to another because that second person is a member of an outgroup that is disrespected by the dominant ingroup. These outgroups include, for example, people of a certain gender, race, or ethnicity; or those with medical symptoms or an illness itself.

The preceding four are by no means an exhaustive list of all the issues around which conflict is generated and negotiation likely to be required. They introduce us, however, to some of the important outcomes that are of value to people and that form the basis of their "interest" and that, when not achieved, serve as a source of disagreement and conflict.

This list of four interests suggests the issues around which negotiation both between individuals and between groups is likely. Unless agreements can be reached in these areas of potential conflict, effective relationships, whether working or personal, are unlikely. Thus, negotiating agreements over money, control, security, and respect is vital if people are to be able to work together. A failure to find a reasonable solution to conflicts in these areas triggers processes that undermine individual and collective well-being.

APPROACHES TO NEGOTIATION

Having established the importance of negotiation as well as some of the issues around which it is likely to take place, we will now examine the ways in which negotiation can be handled. There are skills that can be learned and ways to intervene in a conflict that are helpful for achieving the kind of settlement that will permit the parties to continue functioning together. For the most part, acquiring these skills and intervention strategies is based on learning some of the main concepts about negotiation and mediation.

Kressel and Pruitt (1985) outlined three major categories of interven-tion that are derived from reviewing the literature on mediation. In media-tion, a third party attempts to mediate between two conflicting parties (e.g., two individuals, as in a divorce mediation; two groups, as in labor-management mediation; two nations, as in international mediation). As with any negotiation, the goal of the mediator is to facilitate a settlement and so prevent an escalation of conflict.

In a typical mediation situation, the mediator is not a member of either side and so presumably has the kind of disinterest that members would not possess. Of course, negotiation can occur without a formal outside media-tor. In this case, negotiation would involve the parties who are in disagree-ment. The skills required and the techniques employed are similar, whether one is formally an outside mediator or is a group member taking on this role in order to negotiate a settlement between the conflicting parties.

We have based our own analysis on an adaptation of the Kressel and Pruitt scheme. It includes three points of focus involved in any negotiation situation: individual focus, contextual focus and substantive focus.

The focus on the individual examines those factors within individuals, either within oneself or within others, that may help or hinder a successful negotiation. The focus on the context refers to those factors in the general atmosphere surrounding a conflictive relationship with which a successful negotiator must deal in order to achieve a mutually satisfying solution to the problems that divide the parties. The focus on substantive factors deals most directly with the various strategies that the negotiator might employ in order to help the parties reach a settlement. We will now examine each of these three major categories central to the negotiation process.

INDIVIDUALLY FOCUSED FACTORS
IN NEGOTIATION

As we noted, when we refer to individually focused factors relevant to negotiat-ing a settlement between two parties (e.g., two individuals, two groups), we are concerned with things about the individual person, whether that person is the negotiator or group member, that may either help or hinder the course and the success of a negotiation. We will examine three major themes under this heading: (1) personal styles of negotiating; (2) cognitive biases: (3) bond-ing and establishing trust and rapport.

Personal Styles Of Negotiating

Social psychologists have conducted extensive research in a negotiation situation they have termed the Prisoner's Dilemma (Kelley & Stahelski, 1970; McClintock & Liebrand, 1988; Rapoport & Chammah, 1965; Terhune, 1968). Although it is highly artificial and carried on primarily within the experimenter's laboratory, there are some lessons to be learned from this game about personal styles of negotiating that are relevant to our concerns.

In brief, the Prisoner's Dilemma situation is one in which two persons stand to gain a great deal if they can cooperate, to lose a great deal if each one seeks to maximize her or his own gain, or to achieve a moderate gain if they chose a different strategy. The situation permits us to see an individual's preferred style of negotiation and so gives us some clues that we might be able to use if we are the negotiator or if we find ourselves in a negotiation situation.

In order to create the Prisoner's Dilemma situation, the experimenter establishes a payoff matrix in which one person's actions, when coupled with the actions of the other person, produce a given payoff to each. Consider the following possibility:

		Person A Chooses	
		Red	Black
Person B Chooses	Red	$3/$3	$4/$1
	Black	$1/$4	$1/$1

The dollar amounts in the diagram indicate the money that each person will receive, with Person A's outcome given first in each case. Thus, if Person A chooses Red and Person B also chooses Red, both A and B will receive $3 for this choice. On the other hand, if Person A chooses Black while Person B chooses Red, then Person A will receive $4, whereas Person B will receive only $1. Consider this to be one trial of an experiment in which 30-40 trials could be run with the same two individuals making their choices on each trial.

If you review the situation carefully, you will note that the strategy that would produce the best outcomes for both persons, that is, provide each person with $3, has a risk involved. The risk, of course, is that one person may make a choice that helps her situation but serves to reduce the amount that the other will receive. So, if A chooses Red so that both players will get $3, but B chooses Black so that he will get $4 for himself, the outcome will punish A (who will get only $1), while rewarding B (who will get the desired $4). But what will A do on the next turn? In the situation described, most people settle on the black-black solution, providing a moderate outcome to both, but not the best that they could have achieved together.

The situation as depicted allows for a wide variety of variations: for example, in the payoff amounts, the conditions under which the game is played, and so forth. It is not germane to our present purposes to examine all of these. What we wish to explore at this time, rather, is the interesting finding that people seem to have preferred "styles" of negotiating in this kind of situation. Four main styles have been identified (McClintock & Liebrand, 1988).

The Altruistic Style

The Altruistic Style is one in which individuals are primarily concerned with helping the other party maximize her or his outcomes, disregarding their own outcomes. Clearly, altruism is a self-sacrificing style of negotiating in which people forget their own interests and work only to help others. Of course, it could be argued that helping others is their primary interest, so that the altruistic negotiator feels amply rewarded whenever the other party is rewarded.

Cooperation

Cooperation describes a style in which persons seek to maximize their joint gain (e.g., the $3/$3 outcome). We will shortly examine an approach to attaining this mutually best outcome identified by Axelrod (1984), and indicate some of the conditions under which this cooperative style of negotiating is most likely to work.

Individualism

Individualism refers to a style in which persons attempt to maximize their own payoff, disregarding what the other receives. Individualists, as the term suggests, are fundamentally disinterested in what happens to the other party in the negotiation; as long as they get what they want, they feel satisfied.

Competition

Competition describes a win-lose style in which persons seek to get the most for themselves compared with what others receive. One of the interesting findings about the competitive style, reported some years ago by Kelley and Stahelski (1970), is how this style of negotiating creates a world filled with competitors, thereby vindicating the preference for competition over any other style.

In effect, by relentlessly seeking to conquer the other party, competitors eventually drive others, even those with more cooperative or altruistic styles, to compete. Seeing the other person now competing against them, the competitor feels that it is only correct to do likewise. In other words, competitors justify their own competitiveness by pointing out the competitiveness of other parties, ignoring how their own behavior drove the other parties in that direction in the first place!

While altrusim and cooperation are relatively easy to differentiate, the distinction between the individualistic and competitive negotiating styles might still be somewhat cloudy. In effect, when people come together to resolve the differences that separate them, they have a variety of outcomes they might find acceptable. Individualists are primarily self-focused and concerned less with what others get than with making sure that they get the most they can for themselves. It does not matter to them, therefore, whether others do well or not, only that they themselves do well. By contrast, competitors are concerned precisely with their own relative standing. It matters to them that they come out on top, that they win and someone else loses. They adopt a win-lose worldview. The preferred resolution, therefore requires that they be the winners and that someone else be the loser.

Consider for a moment these negotiating styles in a real-life negotiation situation. Altruists, as defined here, seem to be minimally involved in help-ing advance their own or their group's interests. If one were on the other side, it might be pleasant to have an altruist in the negotiation but it is not readily apparent that one's own group's interests will be met by this style of negotiating. It also seems obvious that neither individualists nor compe-titors will be helpful for creating stable and enduring settlements.

Tit-for-Tat

Cooperation produces the best and most enduring resolution for all parties involved in a negotiation, yet it is not easily accomplished, particu-larly if one is negotiating with individualists or competitors. One form of cooperative strategy, however, that a growing body of research suggests to be valuable, is termed, tit-for-tat: "the strategy that cooperates on the first move and then does whatever the other player did on the previous move" (Axelrod, 1984, p. 20). In other words, a cooperative style employing the tit-for-tat approach would open with a cooperative move and then follow it up with further cooperation—if that is what the other party provides—or with a competitive move—if that is what the other provides. Here is Axelrod's conclusion about the success of this kind of strategy:

> What accounts for Tit-for-Tat's robust success is its combination of being nice, retaliatory, forgiving, and clear. Its niceness prevents it from getting into unneces-sary trouble. Its retaliation discourages the other side from persisting whenever defection is tried. Its forgiveness helps restore mutual cooperation. And its clarity makes it intelligible to the other player, thereby eliciting long-term cooper-ation (p. 54).

McClintock & Liebrand's research (1988) adds to this picture. They find that people consider the person who uses the tit-for-tat strategy to be more intelligent, powerful, fair, and honest than persons who use any of the other styles, even when compared with someone who has adopted a 100 percent cooperative approach. The question, of course, is how to help people involved in negotiation situations learn to adopt a tit-for-tat style rather than sticking to a style that produces less stable and less mutually satisfying agreements.

Axelrod suggests several approaches to increasing the cooperative style, one of the most important of which involves the expansion of people's sense of time. If today's encounter is seen to be the totality of the relationship, then there is little motivation to be cooperative. However, if today's encoun-ter is seen to be part of something more enduring, if people can see that their interactions are not one-shot affairs—but, rather, have an ongoing quality to them—the motivation to cooperate will thereby increase. Axelrod refers to this expanded time sense as "the long shadow of the future." He argues that the sense of the future helps people engage in mutually beneficial cooperation and discourages adopting the less stable and narrowly time-bound strategies of individualism or competition.

Cognitive Factors In Negotiating

In their analysis of mediation, Kressel & Pruitt (1985) refer to one category as "reflexive factors," by which they mean the ways in which people involved in a negotiation orient themselves or, in their words, "fashion themselves into the most effective instrument of conflict management" (p. 188). For our purposes, this focus on the person's preparation for negotiation brings to light the role of cognition in negotiation: that is, how people's ways of thinking and reasoning influence how they negotiate.

Psychologists have demonstrated that the way people process information in a situation influences how they will act in that situation. This is as true for group members as it is for negotiators attempting to work with those members. We have already seen some of these factors at work in our previous discussion of negotiation styles. The competitor enters a situation with a definite win-lose framework of understanding, looking for opportunities to gain the most at another's expense. As we have seen, this is clearly not a helpful manner of approaching a situation that requires negotiation. There are other kinds of cognitive factors that can and do play an important role, particularly a category of "cognitive biases" that people employ when making judgments and reaching decisions.

A variety of cognitive biases have been uncovered in systematic research on this important topic. Most of us will easily recognize how they work.

Self-Fulfilling Prophecy

When we expect something to happen, we often act in very subtle—at times unconscious—ways to make that thing happen. In other words, we fulfill our prophecy. The competitor who created conditions that justified being competitive, in the work we previously mentioned by Kelley and Stahelski, is one such example. There are many other generally known illustrations of this tendency.

Were a traditionally sexist male to interact with a woman, he would do so with the expectation that the woman would be unable to think clearly or make decisions readily, thereby creating a situation that would fulfill his prejudiced expectation. For example, he may interrupt her, make decisions for her in advance, be highly directive, ignore her contributions, and in other ways make it difficult if not impossible for her to act independently. He would then conclude: "See, I'm correct. She is not able to think clearly or independently!"

This kind of cognitive bias could prove disasterous in a negotiation situation. If people were to act based upon their expectations of the other side, they could create the very conditions that would prove the validity of their expectations, rather than having given the other side an opportunity to contradict those expectations. Remember what happens when the competitor defines his or her opponent as another competitor and acts in a manner designed to validate that initial expectation, never giving the other party a chance to cooperate. It is very important for persons who are involved in a negotiation to think through their expectations about the other party and carefully monitor their own behavior so that they do not create the very conditions that fulfill their worst expectations about the other. Let us look at an example of this process at its worst.

A conflict emerged in a large urban hospital between the laboratory and the nursing staff over the proper preparation of patients for laboratory work. Each side blamed the other for failing to act responsibly. Hospital management decided to bring the two sides together to seek a resolution to their conflict. A series of meetings was held comprising representatives of the two groups, management personnel and the hospital's quality control specialist. The quality control specialist, having been trained in group process, observed the initial meetings and quickly sensed that one of the problems preventing resolution of the conflict involved each group's expectations about the other. The laboratory staff, being pressured by the physicians to get lab results completed on an unrealistic time schedule, expected the nurses to side with the physicians rather than being sympathetic to its concerns. This anticipation of hostility led the staff to act in an antagonistic and defensive way toward the nursing staff. Its hostility naturally led the nursing staff to respond in kind, both fulfilling the lab staff's prophecy about the unsympathetic nurses and also creating a condition hardly conducive to working together. In seeing this process at work, the experienced quality control specialist was able to intervene effectively and help the two groups reach an amicable resolution to their conflict.

Other familiar biases involve such tendencies as the following:

1. The tendency to reach a conclusion on an important issue on the basis of the most recently encountered piece of information, ignoring the array of potentially available information (Tversky & Kahneman [1974] termed this the "availability bias"). For example, a supervisor rates her staff's performance based on the most immediately recalled behavior, failing to consider the longer history of its past performance. One nurse who is currently under some stress had not performed as well the day before the evaluation as she had in the past and so was rated lower than others, even though her overall performance had been superior.

2. The tendency to make a judgment on a particular issue using prevailing stereotypes (Tversky & Kahneman termed this the "representativeness bias"). For example, there has been a recent series of airplane crashes and so we

believe it is far more dangerous to fly than to drive, ignoring the reality that driving is far more dangerous than flying.

3. A bias that has been demonstrated to work against two parties seeking to achieve a mutually beneficial agreement involves the tendency that some people have to think in highly simplistic ways (see Tetlock's discussion [1985] of what he refers to as differences in people's integrative complexity). Consider that we may have two extremes. At one end is a negotiation between individuals who have the capability of thinking in complex ways about a situation; at the other, we find simplistically thinking negotiators. The former will be able to take into consideration both their own interests and those of the other party and so arrive at a mutually satisfying compromise. The latter, however, are trapped by their tendency to think only in terms of one side or the other (usually their own), and so tend to having difficulty finding an area of mutually beneficial compromise.

4. Another series of cognitive biases involves our tendency to adopt self-serving views (Greenwald, 1980; Taylor & Brown, 1988), for example, to see ourselves in a more favorable light than is truly warranted. Greenwald argues that these self-serving biases make our ego appear to be totalitarian, designed like a dictator to maintain our ongoing self-aggrandizement in spite of disconfirming information. In his view, however, there are some genuine benefits to the individual who is guarded by the protective shield such biases provide.

Agreeing with Greenwald, Taylor, and Brown suggest that various self-serving illusions (e.g., that we have more control of our lives than we actually have) correlate with good physical and mental health and thus should not be seen as negative. In other words, being somewhat out of touch with reality might actually be good for one's well-being.

While self-serving biases may protect the individual from troublesome information, they may also make a negotiation difficult, especially when people must be open to what the other person wants as well as to their own realistic situation.

The Role Of Bonding In Negotiation

Kressel & Pruitt (1985) mention bonding as one of the central elements in any situation involving mediation and negotiation. Bonding refers to the ways in which people establish rapport with the parties in conflict. Bonding involves establishing trust and, in effect, gaining acceptance. Because it refers to the ways in which the prospective negotiator can act so as to help or hinder the ensuing negotiation, bonding is properly included among the individually focused factors relevant to negotiation.

In general, one of the best ways to bond with others is to "walk in their shoes"—in effect, to begin to see and experience from their perspective. Research on failed negotiations has indicated that the inability to be sensitive to the other person's point of view interferes with successful negotiation (Carroll, Bazerman & Maury, 1988; Tetlock, 1985).

Often in negotiating with others, we focus primarily on our own point of view and what we want to attain. While it is important to keep our own interests clearly in mind, it is also vital to establish a connection with the other party by adopting their perspective and trying to understand their interests. In bonding, we seek connections with the other party that permit a mutually satisfactory resolution to occur because we know where they stand, what they want, and how we appear to them.

Bonding is not an easy accomplishment. It requires both reaching out to the other while simultaneously not losing sight of our own goals and interests. It demands an openness and a receptivity that enables us to listen, hear, and even understand; but it does not require us to accept uncritically. We would certainly not condone the actions of everyone with whom we must negotiate; yet, unless we are able to listen openly to their point of view, we will be unable to achieve the kind of bonding with them that will permit a negotiation to occur.

CONTEXTUAL FACTORS IN NEGOTIATION

The second major category of factors essential in any negotiation involve what we have termed contextual factors (Kressel & Pruitt, 1985). "Contextual factors refer to the mediator's attempts to alter the climate and conditions prevailing between the parties so as to facilitate mutual problem-solving" (Kressel & Pruitt, 1985, p. 191). In this section, we will consider the following factors:

(1) Opening channels of communication between and among the parties;

(2) Helping to diffuse negative perceptions and feelings;

(3) Focusing on the issues;

(4) Structuring an agenda for meetings involving negotiation;

(5) Establishing fair procedures for working together.

Opening Channels Of Communication

Whenever differences between persons or groups arise, one of the first things to occur is a breakdown in communication between the two parties. A breakdown can manifest several ways: people cease to talk with one another; whatever talking that does occur tends to be rather perfunctory; people stop listening to one another; miscommunication and misunderstanding dominate group contacts. Opening the channels of communication, therefore, requires addressing all of these negative possibilities. In effect, to negotiate their differences and achieve some mutually satisfactory agreement, people must begin to talk and listen to each other again. One of the key functions of the negotiator is to help create a climate in which this is possible.

One way to appreciate what is involved in opening channels of communication can be gleaned from considering some of the items used by Thoennes & Pearson (1985) in their study of divorce mediation. They describe the elements that comprise what they refer to as "communication facilitation." They find this factor to be one of the main contributors to successful negotiation between the parties in dispute. Communication facilitation included such items as:

—Helping the parties express their own points of view;
—Helping the parties bring the main issues, problems and feelings to the surface;
—Helping to keep the discussion on track.

Diffusing Negative Perceptions And Feelings

In the typical negotiation situation, the disputing parties may have reached such an antagonistic point in their relationship that one of the prime context-setting tasks involves diffusing the negative perceptions and feelings that abound. It does not help the situation if whenever people talk together all they can experience is "evil" and "anger." When such negative feelings and perceptions dominate, people tend to become defensive and are therefore unable either to advocate on behalf of their own interests or listen to what the other party wants.

Defensiveness harms the negotiation process in two ways. First, we usually become defensive when we feel attacked by the other party. The more defensive we become, the more we lose sight of what it is we have come together to negotiate in the first place. We invest our time and energy into defending and protecting ourselves and into attacking and undermining the other party. Second, if the other party is responding to us in much the same way, it is highly unlikely that any resolution can be achieved. Thus, it is critical to a negotiation that both parties try to diffuse these negative perceptions and feelings.

Diffusing the negative requires redirecting, refocusing, and clarifying—in effect, keeping people away from the hostility and anger. There are several ways to accomplish this, including pointing out to the parties that they are wasting their time together exchanging barbs, rather than talking or listening; redirecting the discussion by ignoring each negative exchange and seeking to focus more clearly on the issues that need to be discussed; engaging in a little humor to break down some of the defensiveness and helping the parties get a better perspective on themselves.

Focusing On The Issues

Conversations in general have a tendency to wander from one topic to another, often with little focus. While some of the delights of interacting together derive from this kind of wandering, it is essential to minimize off-target meandering and help keep the parties more clearly focused on the issues they need to consider when negotiation is the purpose. As noted, keeping the parties focused on the issues also helps deal with some of the problems of negative communication. When we shortly consider some of the substantive factors involved in negotiation, we will return to this same point involving focusing.

Structuring An Agenda

It is important to set an agenda for any meeting that involves negotiation including preplanning as opposed to ongoing guidance of conversation. An agenda helps structure the task the parties confront and helps direct them away from angry outbursts and toward the reason they have convened in the first place. An agenda also helps minimize the frustration we all feel at many meetings we attend that seem to go nowhere. An agenda makes it clear that certain goals are to be reached during this meeting and thereby allows people to evaluate their progress toward those goals.

An agenda also helps a group chart a series of negotiating sessions rather than assuming that everything must be settled all at once. One session is usually insufficient to complete all the negotiating tasks that are required. The impatience that people feel can be reduced by showing that today's task was only attempting to get from point A to point C; that the next meeting will begin with B in the hopes of moving forward to E, and so forth.

Finally, an agenda provides the very kind of structure that helps reduce the anxiety we all feel when confronting a relatively open horizon of possibilities without boundaries to contain us. Containing the anxiety that stems from a lack of structure is especially important in negotiation for some of the reasons we have previously considered, (e.g., diffusing negative communication, keeping people focused on their tasks).

Establishing Fair Procedures

One of the prime requirements of any negotiation is that the parties experience the environment within which they are working together to be functioning in a fair manner. If things seem to be leaning in favor of one side or the other, this kind of imbalance will suggest that no reasonable outcome is possible. In some cases, procedural fairness may be as or more vital than the actual outcomes that issue from the negotiation (Tyler, 1987).

For example, if one person wins something and another loses something as the result of a negotiation, the way that outcome is evaluated may be a function of the fairness of the procedures that led to that result. If the procedures are perceived to be fair, then the outcomes—even if they provide more benefits to one group over another—may be more acceptable. Conversely, if the procedures by which the outcomes were achieved are not perceived as being fair, whatever outcomes were accomplished will be undermined.

One of the most important elements that help make a procedure fair involves having a genuine voice in the discussion and in the shaping of outcomes. When people feel themselves deprived of their "voice," they are sure to consider any outcomes unfair. Admittedly, a personally beneficial outcome that happens to be granted to one of the parties may initially seem fair to the advantaged party. On reflection, however, if we can be granted benefits by someone else without having a voice in this determination, it follows that the same individual can also undo those benefits to our detriment. It is better, then, to have voice in the procedures that benefit or harm us than to be at the capricious mercy of someone else.

In a culture in which the adversarial process is employed extensively for resolving disputes, it is hardly surprising that many people have come to believe that an adversarial process is the guarantor of fair procedure in other areas of life as well. This belief can be helpful to a negotiation because it tells us that the determination of right and wrong is held in abeyance until all parties have had an opportunity to present their side.

The belief in the procedural legitimacy of an adversarial process can also be helpful in suggesting that what should properly occur between the disputing parties is a hearing in which each side gets to present its perspective and in which challenges are proper.

Unlike the law courts or formal mediation, however, there is no judge or jury standing outside to render a verdict in most negotiations. Therefore, in negotiation, procedural fairness that is based on a belief in the adversarial system has no simple set of external standards to employ for reaching a final accord. Insofar as people believe that the adversarial procedure is fair, however, at least the negotiated outcome stands a reasonably good chance of being acceptable on procedural grounds.

An example of what we mean by procedural fairness involves a case of its violation when the Director of Nursing asked her nursing staff to participate in a decision that had already been made. While it initially appeared to the nursing staff that it had "voice" in the decision process, the facts were very different. When the nurses learned that the decision had already been made, they felt duped by the Director of Nursing who had invited their participation in a situation in which it was not real. In responses to their justified anger, the Director became very defensive, declining to meet with her staff to discuss the issues, adding further to an already strained situation. We return to fill out the details of this example in Chapter 12.

SUBSTANTIVE FACTORS IN NEGOTIATION

Up to this point, we have been considering individual and contextual factors that are relevant to the process of negotiation. As we now consider the final category of factors, the substantive, we trust that it is clear that we have divided the territory of negotiation into three parts as a convenience to help clarify the negotiation process, not because these are independent. Kressel & Pruitt (1985) define the substantive factors involved in negotiation as "those tactics by which the mediator deals directly with the issues in dispute. These tactics aim to narrow the gap and precipitate a settlement" (p. 192). We will consider five substantive issues: (1) rivals and constituents; (2) trade-offs; (3) areas of overlap; (4) power; and (5) the future.

Rivals And Constituents

Since none of us lives in a vacuum, our negotiating with another party is usually significantly influenced by all of our relationships with others who are not immediately present at the negotiation. There are two kinds of significant others who may affect what kind of concessions we feel we can make with the other party: our rivals and our constituents.

The point we are making is that the two parties involved in a negotiation are not the only participants relevant to the outcome. Rivals, those who stand to benefit from our failures, are always in the wings, watching and waiting. We are usually aware of their presence and perhaps of their eagerness to see us fare poorly so that they can step in and benefit. We may therefore be unable to make certain concessions in a given negotiation because we fear the benefit this will provide our rivals.

One sees this process occurring in labor-management negotiations in which, for example, Hospital N's settlement with its striking nurses may put that hospital at a competitive disadvantage compared to other hospitals in its area. Hospital N's negotiators are thereby reluctant to make certain concessions to its own nursing staff lest the rival hospitals use them to their own benefit.

Of course, the nursing staff at the rival hospitals have a stake in the settlement reached by the nurses at Hospital N. Not only are these other nurses part of the constituency of the nursing staff negotiating at Hospital N, but their presence may help achieve agreements at Hospital N that would not otherwise be possible. Likewise, the settlement they observe nurses at Hospital N achieving might fuel their own later bargaining sessions with their own hospital's administrators.

As this example illustrates, in addition to our rivals' anticipating poor outcomes for us, we also have constituents in the wings rooting for us because our outcomes will effect theirs. Our awareness of the constituency also helps shape what we feel we can and cannot do within a given negotiation.

The preceding suggests that negotiation is a complex matter. Not only must the immediate participants be considered, and a resolution sought that is mutually satisfactory to them, but the process and the resolution must also be something that each party can live within light of the demands of both their rivals and their constituents. Because of their importance to the negotiation process, it is usually necessary to have a direct discussion of rivals and constituents within the negotiation itself.

International relations offers us several further illustrations of this point. We often see one side permitting the other side with whom it is in negotiation to posture and to adopt an extreme position, in full knowledge that this is being done for the audience back home and has very little to do with the actual negotiating between the disputing parties.

The preceding point is an important one and should be carefully considered. We may have to allow the persons with whom we are engaged in a negotiation to act in ways that publicly help them deal with both their rivals and their constituents, while discounting the importance of this posturing for the actual negotiation in which we are involved with them. If we deny them this opportunity (or if they deny it to us), we may find it impossible to reach agreements which require concessions on both sides.

Trade-offs

To negotiate is to make concessions. This means that neither we nor the other party get everything that each wants. We each get something, but also must make a variety of concessions to the other side in the name of reaching a satisfactory settlement. The idea of a trade-off is a helpful way of formulating this issue: we see that a concession in one area is traded for a desired outcome in another. If we consider a concession to be the loss of something we value, we may decline to make concessions. This will not help a negotiation that, by definition, requires concessions all around. By making a concession part of a package—giving up one benefit in order to get another—we may be more willing to make the concession.

The ideas of concessions and of trade-offs are essential elements of any negotiation. The parties to a negotiation need to be made aware of these ideas early in the process if a negotiation is to be successful. Negotiations will proceed more effectively if persons are aware of the two concepts (concessions and trade-offs) and have also carefully thought through and evaluated their own situation so that they know their limits and what they are willing to concede.

If the nature of the dispute separating the parties is grounded on deeply held principles that are in conflict, it may not, of course, be possible to find trade-offs. Yet, unless a negotiation is entered with a willingness to give a little in order to get something, it has no chance to succeed.

Areas Of Overlap

Rarely are the parties involved in a negotiation at such extreme positions that they have little in common to begin the process of dialogue in the first place. One of the important early tasks of any negotiation, therefore, is to chart areas of substantial overlap and agreement between the parties. This charting will not only help the parties feel better about one another by seeing their commonalities, but will also help establish a basis for making the necessary concessions and trade-offs that will appear in the negotiated settlement they eventually reach.

Overlap in long-term goals, for example, can prove very beneficial to a negotiation. We may have a situation, as noted in several previous examples, in which physicians and nursing staff disagree about a particular procedure and must negotiate some mutually satisfactory agreement. One clear area of overlap is their shared concern for quality health care. While they may disagree about some of the particulars, this goal stands out as a central feature of overlap between them as well as a helpful theme to surface repeatedly when the negotiation session becomes overly tense.

Several ideas should be kept in mind when seeking to chart areas of overlap between the disputing parties. It is important to explore areas of potential compromise—issues around which there is minimal disagreement and therefore around which resolution can be reached—early in the process. Leave those areas that continue to separate the parties until later in the process, framing them in the context of the many substantial agreements already reached.

It is also relevant for the negotiator to take an active role in suggesting possible agreements and areas of overlap that might have escaped the protagonists' attention. This requires carefully listening to both sides and working to develop a list of commonalities to present back to each party. Finally, it is also helpful for the negotiator to assist the parties in analyzing the pros and the cons of the several tentative resolutions to their disagreement that begin to appear. This proves to be important in that it can increase areas of overlap and also highlight points that continue to require attention.

Power

In many negotiation situations, one party occupies a position of greater power than another by virtue of their position in the organizational heirarchy. Three unhelpful outcomes of this difference in power are possible. First, the more powerful might arrogantly seek to use its power to force a settlement. Second, the less powerful might feel so intimidated that it fails to advocate on behalf of its own interests and so concedes from the outset. Third, the less powerful might become so excessively belligerent that it makes demands that are virtually impossible for the more powerful to concede.

A substantial body of research suggests that those holding less power in a negotiation situation, in fact, have much more power than they might imagine. Therefore, they neither have to yield everything to the more powerful nor press forward to engage the more powerful in the kind of battle that the less powerful can rarely win (Moscovici, 1985). A consistently held position, argued forcefully can, over time, affect the more powerful, compelling them to make concessions that they might not have otherwise have thought necessary.

World history offers us numerous instances of the powerful oppressing minorities, only to find themselves undermined and having to yield in the face of a continued refusal of the minorities to remain oppressed. The course of influence does not always run in a direction that favors the powerful. Minorities can, and will, continue to operate traffic in both directions, influencing those who seek to influence them and winning concessions that they might never have imagined possible when they first entered into the negotiation.

The Future

One of the most important outcomes of any negotiation is the way it establishes a foundation for future relationships between the parties. If a disagreement is resolved in such a way that bad feelings remain, it is not likely that future relationships among the parties who must continue working together will be healthful. As we saw earlier in considering Axelrod's recommendations regarding cooperation, if that future course is kept well in mind, it may contribute to the resolution of the current dispute. If that future is ignored, the current situation may be resolved but will not be helpful to either establish an ongoing working relationship or a process for future negotiation.

Thus, there are two aspects of the future that are important to keep in mind: (1) When people must continue to work and live together, settlements reached today must include consideration of the continued relationship of the parties involved. Thus, winning by demeaning or destroying the other party is not helpful. That party is not likely to forget! (2) When people must continue to work and live together, the future is also relevant in that the manner in which the current dispute is resolved provides a basis for resolving future disputes. A negotiating process today that is evaluated positively by all involved will lay a solid foundation for future negotiations.

SUMMARY AND CONCLUSIONS

This chapter has attempted to present the sometimes complex but vital picture of negotiation that is involved in interpersonal, intragroup, and intergroup processes. We have provided a summary chart of the topics, issues, and themes we have presented in Table 10-1.

Table 10-1. Negotiation Issues and Strategies

I.   Individually Focused Factors

    A. Negotiating Styles

       1. altruistic

       2. individualistic

       3. cooperative

     4. competitive

  B. Cognitive Factors and Biases

     1. self-fulfilling prophecy

     2. availability bias

     3. representativeness bias

     4. integrative complexity

     5. self-serving biases

  C. Bonding

II. Contextual Factors

  A. Opening Channels of Communication

  B. Diffusing Negative Feelings and Perceptions

  C. Focusing on Issues

  D. Structuring an Agenda

  E. Establishing Fair Procedures

III. Substantive Factors

  A. Rivals and Constituents

  B. Trade-Offs

  C. Areas of Overlap

  D. Power

  E. The Future

We have provided a useful overview of the strategies that one must employ, whether seeking to negotiate with a friend over a personal issue, a co-worker over a work issue or organizational representatives over employment issues.

All of us are, in fact, involved in a variety of negotiations everyday in our personal and our work lives, although we may hesitate to refer to these as negotiations. Invariably, however, we are always seeking a mutually satisfactory course of action with the people with whom we work, the people we supervise, our employers, our patients, and our clients. By considering these exchanges as negotiations and by allowing the negotiation process to involve the various issues and strategies presented in this chapter—and summarized in Table 10-1—we hope to have improved the skills with which this common process is undertaken and to thereby improve the degree to which mutually satisfactory resolutions are possible.

11

Observation and Diagnosis

*I*t is axiomatic to state that before health professionals can work effectively with groups, they must be able to assess and to evaluate the critical characteristics of group structure and process previously considered. In this chapter, we will introduce some of the general observational approaches involved in this assessment.

All of us function within groups; many thereby believe themselves to be intuitively expert about how groups function. However, it takes training and experience to properly and confidently assess this world of our everyday group interactions. In fact, it is the very common sense quality of our social world that erroneously leads many to believe themselves to possess expertise without need for further direction or training.

We practice what one psychologist has referred to as "bubbapsychology" (McGuire, 1969), using the timeworn homilies of our grandmothers to deal with others. Unfortunately, those intuitive, grandmotherly bits of advice may guide us in opposite directions. For example, one piece of advice to a parent or a group leader suggests that if you "spare the rod you will spoil the child." However, we also learn that "you can catch more flies with honey than with vinegar." So, should the leader be stern and harsh or sweet and kindly? Grandma never tells us everything.

The same bubbapsychology can lead us astray as well when it comes to assessing group process. What are we to conclude when we look at a group of people some of whom are talking, sometimes all at once; others of whom are silent, sometimes all at once? It is difficult enough to know what to look for or at when we attend to one person. But a group ... ? What we need to develop is a knowledge of some of the major concepts and approaches to group observation that we can systematically employ to sharpen our understanding and to make our intuitive, personal experiences more useful for our daily practice.

OBSERVATION VS. INTERPRETATION

The best tools health professionals possess for assessing groups are their own eyes and ears. It will be helpful to examine some of the general approaches available for observing group and individual behavior. But first, note that we are referring to *systematic* observation. This is to emphasize the point that it is best to observe according to some system rather than in a haphazard or casual manner. We separate what we see or hear from the inferences and interpretations we make based on these observations. For example, we see a smile and infer happiness. We attempt to record and note actual behaviors. We employ known systems for our observations or develop our own systematic framework for the particular purposes at hand.

The point is critical. It is important for observers to be able to separate what they actually see or hear from what they interpret that observation to mean. We do not see anger as such; we do see various behaviors that can lead us to infer anger. For example, Dr. Jones raises his voice above its previous conversational level. He clenches his hands and appears to make a fist. He moves about in his chair, pushing it back from the table; his gestures become larger and more expansive. His face reddens somewhat and his lips become tight. As we listen to *what* he says, we note that the content involves his defense of an intern's right to observe a special procedure even before there has been a detailed study of it. A legitimate inference is that Dr. Jones is angry.

One of the best ways for students to develop their own ability to separate observations from interpretations and to insure that they will be systematic rather than casual about this process is to use a recording form such as the following:

Behaviors Seen or Heard	*Interpretations and Inferences*
1. M. smiles.	1. M. is happy.
2. Dr. Jones raises his voice; clenches his fist; makes large gestures; speaks in defense of an intern.	2. Dr. Jones is angry.

One of the clear advantages to working with such a format is that it gives observers a record of the actual behaviors on which they based their inferences. No comparable record would exist if observers simply recorded interpretations but failed to systematically present the behavioral data on which those were based. Without this record, it is not possible for someone else to evaluate the observations; nor is it possible to test and validate an analysis.

Often it is necessary to gather observations over time in order to test and confirm or disprove an interpretation of behavior. When these observations have been systematically obtained the interpretations can be tested; preliminary analyses can be reevaluated in the light of later observations. This cannot be done, however, if there is no systematic listing of actual observations separated from early or preliminary interpretations.

Let us take an example to sharpen this point. Recall Families, Inc., a group practice that was first introduced in Chapter 1. Imagine we are sitting in during one of their meetings at which they are reviewing a particularly difficult case. One member of the practice, an R.N. is relatively new to the group and to nursing as well. When she speaks during the meetings, her voice is very soft and difficult to hear; she uses many pauses and "uh" sounds that typically suggest anxiety (Kasl & Mahl, 1965). She sits back in her chair, almost withdrawing physically from the others in the group. Most of what she says indicates agreement with whatever anyone else in the group has been saying. We record these observations and make our initial interpretation: "Nurse Smith appears to be anxious, not surprising for someone new to nursing and to this group practice; she seems to us to be eager to please and to gain acceptance into the group." Because we are aware of her newness to the profession and to this practice, we may feel very confident about our interpretations, appreciating the difficulties that anyone who is a recent graduate and undertaking her first real work in a setting such as this is likely to experience.

We continue to observe the group's interaction. Later in the same session, we observe the same nurse. Now her manner is more vocal. She speaks much more loudly and in rapid bursts; the pace of her speech has picked up considerably. She has lost the hesitations that characterized her initial conversations. She leans forward in her chair; her gestures have become larger and more expansive. What she says has also changed. She now openly argues and disagrees with the others. Our interpretation as we now observe her is that Nurse Smith seems angry and upset with the group.

We now have a listing of two sets of observations and two somewhat disparate interpretations. We still do not have enough material on which to base a conclusion; we do, however, have a relatively firm base of behavioral observations on which to test out one of the competing analyses of Nurse Smith's behavior. Several possibilities exist. We could test each interpretation by directly intervening and asking her a question: e.g., "I've noticed that your manner has changed from early in this session when you spoke hesitantly and sat back in your chair to the present, when you are speaking more forcefully and even argumentatively. I was wondering what this change might mean." Or we might decide to gather more behavioral observations in order to confirm or disprove one of these interpretations or even to develop a different analysis of her behavior and its meaning.

Whichever approach we adopt, it is important to note that they are both built upon our having first systematically distinguished between observations and interpretations. This has permitted us to recall to Nurse Smith her actual behaviors as well as our interpretations and thereby to provide her some behavioral basis for our intervention. This has also provided us with a listing of behaviors and preliminary interpretations that we now have available for later confirmation or refutation.

Types of Observational Data

Basically, there are two types of material available for systematic observation: nonverbal and verbal. Nonverbal observation deals with the mannerisms, gestures, spatial arrangements, touching, intonation, and other such qualities of a person's or a group's behavior. Verbal observation involves both the actual *content* of what is said and the *forms* by which the communication occurs. Content involves what is said, what the people are actually talking about. Form has to do with word choices, use of language (e.g., colloquial or more formal and/or technical), address forms that are used, and so forth. For purposes of assessing group process, we are interested in all of these sources of information. We will begin our analysis with a consideration of the observation of nonverbal behavior.

OBSERVING NONVERBAL BEHAVIORS

Even in our silences we communicate. We who spend so much of our lives talking and trying to choose our words carefully, too often forget the critical role that nonverbal behavior plays in communicating with others. Verbal behavior tends to be more readily under a person's control than the less easily managed nonverbal forms of communication. Sensitive observation of the nonverbal, therefore, can be a potent assessment tool for understanding individual and group process.

Perhaps no profession is more engaged in the observation of nonverbal behavior than the medical and health professions. Persons are taught to observe the slightest change in skin color, for example, as an indicator of possible respiratory disorder. Health professionals note restlessness, body posture, hand gestures, and voice quality (e.g., intonation) to help clarify their medical diagnosis. How often, however, do health professionals observe these nonverbal behaviors in order to determine psychological and interpersonal functioning? Much can be learned about individuals' psychological state (e.g., Are they anxious, depressed, angry?) and about a group's interpersonal state (e.g., Is group morale high or low? Is the group cohesive? Is there conflict within the group?) through observations of nonverbal behavior. For convenience, it is possible to map out several types of nonverbal behavior that are open to our systematic observation and analysis. These include tactile, proxemic, kinesic, and paralinguistic.

Tactile

Tactile communication involves the sense of touch. Individuals as well as cultures vary extensively in their use of touching in communicating. In the United States, for example, males usually do not embrace as a form of greeting; in many Eastern European and Latin American cultures, on the other hand, the embrace between males is not unusual (Jourard, 1968). Some families are high in their tactile communication—children are frequently held, caressed, and touched by parents; family members walk together arm in arm, embrace during times of sorrow and times of great joy. Other families, by contrast, rarely physically touch—children learn to avoid touching other than the few formal gestures, such as handshakes, that most of us have learned. Anyone involved with patient care realizes that touching can be a potent form of reassurance; withholding this type of body contact may communicate an uncaring or disinterested attitude.

In medicine, patients are constantly being physically touched by doctors, nurses, aides, and attendants. The most intimate body parts are manipulated by hand and instrument often in a painful and intrusive manner. The way in which the professional touches the patient can communicate hurry, harassment, disinterest, embarrassment, insecurity, incompetence; or concern, caring, reassurance, competence. A patient may rapidly lose confidence in the professional who tactually communicates inexperience in contrast to the more experienced hand.

Tactile communication within a group may be used by the leader as an intervention or to develop an analysis of the status of the group or its members. In the former, the leader may hold or touch a member who is experiencing difficulty or rejection as a gesture of comfort, support, or reassurance. In the latter, the leader-observer may use tactile communication to assess the feeling-tone (e.g., cohesiveness and closeness among members) of the group. A great deal of touching can be an indicator that a group is concerned and cares for its members, that it seeks to provide much support and reassurance. Little touching can indicate a lack of concern, a climate of impersonality or formality. Naturally any interpretations based on these observations must take into consideration a range of other factors in addition to touching per se: e.g., the setting, the culture, the sex of the participants, and so forth.

There is some interesting research, for example, that reports differences between men and women and between high and low status individuals in their use of touching to communicate (Henley, 1977). It has been shown that men tend to touch women more than women touch men and that high-status persons in a group tend to touch low-status individuals more than vice versa. It is likely that these findings are linked, insofar as in myriad work settings, women tend to occupy lower status positions than men. It may therefore be that men touch women more because men occupy high-status positions in which touching of low-status employees is more likely to occur than the reverse.

Henley reports other findings involving status differences in nonverbal behavior that go beyond touch and enter the arena of the other categories of nonverbal behavior that we will be considering. For example, as compared with persons occupying higher status positions within a group or organization, low-status individuals tend to smile more, nod more, have a more rigid posture, and keep both their arms and legs close to their bodies when speaking. Recall some of our observations of Nurse Smith from a previous example;

some of her nonverbal behavior suggested her sense of herself as occupying a lower status in this group, at least initially.

Proxemics

Proxemics involves the study of communication by and through the use of space. The early research on animals' defense of territory provided the impetus for parallel studies of human territoriality. In particular, a concern has been directed toward studying conversation distances that persons use for formal and informal interaction (Hall, 1959; 1963; Little, 1968). Research has suggested a cultural variation in this distance; in some cultures, for example, standing breath-to-breath for all conversations is considered appropriate. This often confuses the cultural alien who is used to having greater distance (e.g., 3 feet) between self and others. Violating this distance breaks the implicit shield some people carry around themselves, often creating unintended messages. For example, if 3 to 5 feet in distance is considered comfortable for a typical conversation in the United States, then whenever persons stand either closer or farther away, they are communicating something beyond the usual. Excessive closeness may communicate greater intimacy than is desired; distance may indicate a wish to break off the interaction by taking leave.

Sometimes group members move their chairs closely together as a mood of warmth and camaraderie takes over during a meeting. The keen observer of proxemics can determine much about the cohesiveness of a group by noting the arrangement of chairs during or after a meeting. Subgroup formation may likewise often be determined by simply noting which individuals spatially cluster together and how much distance separates them from other subgroups.

An intervention technique usefully employed in some types of groups actually builds upon proxemic communication. The technique involves placing a marker in the center of the room (e.g., a piece of paper or an X to mark the center). Members are asked to consider that center mark as being the ideal group member or the most ideal group they can imagine. Members are then asked to locate themselves around that marker, using their distance from it to indicate how closely they feel they approximate the ideal. After persons have arranged themselves, the leader then asks each to talk about why they located themselves as they did, how others feel about each person's location, and what steps would be needed to move each person closer in toward that ideal spot.

This technique often reveals a great deal about the group. For example, it can reveal subgroup formations as some members cluster themselves together and separated from others. It can reveal members who feel themselves separate from the group—some may actually locate themselves outside the meeting room or at the doorway. Proxemics can be a useful tool to determine group members' feelings about the group or about their function within the group.

Compensation

A principle of *compensation* has been noted by some analysts of prox-emic behavior (Argyle & Dean, 1965; Patterson, 1968). When an individual stands too close for comfort, there is a tendency for the other person to com-pensate by averting the eyes, leaning backwards, or by presenting a side rather than a straight-on body orientation. On the other hand, when someone stands beyond the comfort range, compensation involves the other person's lean-ing forward and staring more directly into the other's eyes.

Immediacy Cues

One investigator, Mehrabian (1971), has introduced the concept of immediacy cues to refer to a set of nonverbal, primarily proxemic (but includ-ing kinesic as well) information that communicates the *degree of liking or dis-liking that is involved in a relationship.* Immediacy cues involve distance, body orientation, and eye gaze. Thus, if a person stands at some distance from another, orients his or her body away from that person, and tends not to look at the other, the message of dislike or of impersonality may well be non-verbally communicated. Note that the person may not have consciously intended this message; nevertheless, the receiver picks up the message and may respond accordingly.

Impressions

Many of our impressions of others are derived on the basis of their non-verbal behavior; their impressions of us are likewise influenced by our non-verbal as well as our verbal messages. Clearly, the observer of group process must become sensitive to members' nonverbal behavior in order to under-stand what is going on. For example, normative pressures may be communi-cated nonverbally; deviant members are rejected proxemically, for example, by other members locating themselves at some distance or refusing to inter-act with a more friendly, face-to-face body orientation.

Likewise, the observer may note that a member communicates her atti-tude proxemically, by the way in which she locates herself spatially in the group. A member may express anger, for example, by physically separating herself from other group members. Or another may be communicating dis-interest or boredom by leaning back or away from the rest of the group. The observer must be sensitive to this form of information, especially, for exam-ple, when a member's opinions have been criticized and he physically with-draws from further participation. The use of space communicates to the observer and others that person's feeling or rejection; he says *spatially* what he feels. This observation may motivate the observer-leader to intervene to help bring the member back into the group or to help him deal with his feelings of rejection.

The implications for the practicing health professional are critical. When we realize how much our impressions of patients and their impressions of us derives from nonverbal proxemic information, and in turn, how those impressions can seriously influence the success of our practice, we must reassess this mode of our communication. For example, the dying patient often first becomes aware of this prognosis when the nurses proxemically (and inadvertently) communicate it to them. Although they use reassuring words, their spatial separation and avoidance speaks to the patient much louder than anything they say verbally.

Status and Proxemics

Proxemic communication involves many complex interpersonal issues. Sommer's work (1969) has been especially instructive in showing how persons arrange the spatial features in a room or at a table in order to communicate something to others. For example, people who wish to be left alone may communicate this desire nonverbally by locating themselves at the end of a rectangular table; or they may place themselves squarely in the center, surrounded by territorial markers (e.g., coats, books, etc.) to communicate "this is my table and I don't want anyone else to sit nearby."

Power and status are likewise communicated spatially: sitting behind a large desk facing the patient and others from behind its protective barrier emphasizes formality of relationship between persons of differing power and status. Proxemic messages are used extensively in small groups. People who wish to adopt the leadership position within the group may literally situate themselves spatially so as to be at the group's center or at its spatial focal point.

Kinesics

Kinesic communication primarily involves a language of gestures, including movements of the body, limbs, the face, and especially the eyes. There has been an extensive array of research attempting to uncover the meanings of body language. There is much debate concerning whether or not persons universally express themselves kinesically in the same way, or if there are culture and situation-specific modes of kinesic communication. For example, is anger universally expressed by the same facial gestures or do these vary by culture? For the observer of group process, it is less important to resolve such an issue than to be able to recognize and become proficient in noting how others use their bodies and their eyes to communicate. Kinesic communication provides a rich source of information about persons' feelings and thoughts and about the kinds of relationships that emerge when two or more people interact.

Leakage

Paul Ekman's work has been especially enlightening regarding the importance of kinesic communication (Ekman, 1964; I965a; b; Ekman & Friesen, 1969; 1974; Ekman, et al., 1972). One investigation suggested the principle of *nonverbal leakage*. Ekman believed that individuals are more in control of facial and head cues than bodily cues, and thus the body is more likely than the head to "leak" real feelings. To study this, Ekman filmed individuals who were intentionally being deceptive about their true feelings, trying to hide them from others. He showed these films to several groups, some of whom saw only the deceiver's head, others only the body, and still others the full person. Ekman's expectation that the body would show the true feelings better than the head was substantiated. People who had seen either the full individual or the body were more accurate in surmising that person's deception than were those who saw only the head. The implication for the practitioner is obvious; if we have reason to believe that people are intentionally trying to deceive us or even that they may be ignorant of their own real feelings, we can learn a great deal by attending to body gestures that "leak" these feelings.

MMEs

Additional research reported by Ekman demonstrated the importance of what he termed *micromomentary expressions* (MME). These refer to rather small movements of muscle groups in the face. Some of these movements are so tiny, in fact, that the typical viewer can discern them easily only when they have been filmed and the film is shown at a very slow speed. Yet there are some people who seem capable of noting these MMEs even during interaction, suggesting an important individual difference in the capability of perceiving nonverbal kinesic behavior. We return to this issue of individual differences shortly.

Attention to MMEs can offer the observer further information about the feelings and attitudes of others. A patient, for example, may verbally express little concern about a forthcoming surgical procedure; perhaps in our own eagerness to avoid dealing with his or her tension, we accept that person's verbal message at face value and probe no further. However, the keen observer may note the patient's more subtle gestures (i.e., MMEs) that inform us of anxiety and tension. Such practitioners are now better equipped to help the patient; they have recognized the tension expressed nonverbally and thus can work more effectively with the patient before surgery.

Eyes

Kinesics also involves movements of the hands and the eyes. The eyes are especially informative. Exline and his associates demonstrated how either excessive or too little eye contact between persons can be discomforting (Exline, 1971). Some research showed, for example, how 0 percent or 100 percent eye contact was less comfortable than eye contact in the 50 percent range. Thus, people who stare relentlessly at others may inadvertently communicate in ways that cause them to be disliked or feared; their excessive eye contact may increase tension and aversion in others.

Other investigations have suggested that people seem to prefer more eye contact when the communication is positive and less when it is negative (Ellsworth & Carlsmith, 1968). The power implications of eye contact have also been demonstrated. Exline's work suggested a tendency for those low in power to look more at those in high power than vice versa. Furthermore, persons who are seeking to establish dominance in a relationship are thought to attempt to "capture" the other's gaze.

Once again, we can readily note the implications of these findings for the observer of group process as well as for the practitioner. Observers can use their assessment of eye contact within group interaction, for example, as one way of evaluating the power relationships that exist or are being sought: e.g., who tries to capture other's glances; who is looked at most frequently.

We have noticed in some of our own work with groups, for example, that certain members will frequently look at the leader. They seem forever trying to examine the leader as though to determine what he or she is thinking. One interpretation of this observation is that such members may be insecure and are seeking approval and direction from the person in authority. Of course, this is not the only interpretation possible, but it is one that warrants consideration and attempts to validate: e.g., "I've noticed that you frequently look at me. I'm not sure what this means or what you want, but I have the feeling that you are waiting for me to do something or to say something."

Leadership

Another substantial contribution to kinesic communication has been made by Birdwhistell (1952), who observed how leadership in a group of adolescent boys was communicated kinesically rather than verbally. An observer of the boys' verbal behavior would note little difference between the group's leader and other members with respect to initiating conversations or frequency of participation. However, group leaders were noted to be "kinesically more mature" than group members. They engaged in less fidgeting, less foot shuffling, fewer extraneous movements. Furthermore, posturally, they were especially good and attentive listeners: that is, their gestural language communicated interest in, concern for, and attention to others in their group. Their leadership was communicated primarily through their nonverbal, kinesic movements rather than by what they said or how frequently they said it.

Hands

Hand movements, in particular hand rubbing, has come under the scrutiny of another team of investigators concerned with kinesic behavior (Freedman, Blass, Rifkin & Quitkin, 1973). That research demonstrated a fascinating link between hand movements and verbal behavior. Specifically, it was found that during periods in which the individual was covertly hostile and angry, hand movements peaked. During periods of direct, overt hostility, hand rubbing decreased and hand movements tended to be used more to emphasize the verbal hostility (e.g., the hands were used to punctuate the anger that was being overtly expressed verbally.) The keen observer may be able to determine another's attitudes and feelings by watching their hand movements rather than depending solely on their verbal communication.

Paralinguistics

The final category of nonverbal communication involves paralinguistic behavior—verbalizations that are not, strictly speaking, words. These include intonations, pauses, pitch, intensity, the use of such sounds as "uh-huh," and so forth. Kasl and Mahl's research (1965) has demonstrated an important link between tension and the excessive use of "uh" and similar utterances. The trained practitioner can become sensitive to paralinguistic signs of tension or anxiety: e.g., the client's voice may crack, his or her pace may quicken, pauses may lengthen, intonation may flatten. The latter is especially informative about depression.

Paralinguistics provides the observer with a rich source of information about group feelings as well as individual feelings. An entire group may demonstrate boredom on the one hand or involvement or anxiety on the other through paralinguistic means. Long, rambling, and monotonously intoned conversations within the group, for example, might inform the leader that involvement and interest are low. This should motivate a search for possible reasons: e.g., perhaps group members are bored and disinterested because they are unclear about their purposes or goals, or because the task is one that was designed for them by the leader rather than the one that they agreed to do. Rapidly paced, quick bursts of conversation or conversation that is high-pitched and intense can indicate either excitement or anxiety in the group. Further observations of other kinds of verbal and nonverbal material are required to determine which of these is present: e.g., we are likely to affirm an interpretation of anxiety rather than joyful excitement if we also observe some members' physical withdrawal, hear and see rapid breathing, hear content that involves difficulties, tensions, and conflict.

INDIVIDUAL DIFFERENCES IN
NONVERBAL BEHAVIOR

As has been noted, there are cultural as well as individual differences in nonverbal behavior. Individual differences within the same general cultural group are especially important to understand. Ekman's research suggested that although some people appear to be more sensitive to MMEs than others, most people can be trained to develop sensitivity to microexpressions. A kind of intuitive "feeling" for the moods and feelings of others may reflect a high sensitivity. It is possible to train individuals to develop more empathy as they develop their abilities to observe and to be responsive to nonverbal communications.

Senders

Another type of critical individual difference pertains less to the receiver or observer of the nonverbal behavior than to the sender. Some important experimental research has demonstrated, for example, a rather striking difference between males and females in their abilities as senders of nonverbal messages (Buck, et al., 1974). Teams were composed with one person assigned the role of sender and the other the role of receiver (i.e., observer). Each sender was given some pictures to examine while the receiver observed the nonverbal, primarily facial responses to these pictures from an adjoining room. The receiver's task was simply to identify the picture that the sender was examining entirely on the basis of nonverbal facial cues. Teams with male senders did less well than teams with female senders. In other words, the ability to accurately read another person's nonverbal behavior, in this instance, appeared to be a function of individual variations in the ability to clearly send nonverbal messages, rather than a function of the training of the observer.

If we may generalize beyond these findings, the implication is that some persons provide us with less helpful nonverbal indicators of their feelings and attitudes than do others. Yet even here the data emphasize facial communication. The range of nonverbal cues we have noted is substantial; the observer may be able to determine ways in which poor facial senders communicate through other channels. At least, the trained observer-practitioner would not expect his or her male clients (or male group members) to be as helpful in their facial nonverbal indications as their female clients; thus the observer-practitioner would do well to become more attentive to other channels of nonverbal communication that may be informative for males.

VERBAL VS. NONVERBAL BEHAVIOR

According to Bateson and others, all communication contains two levels of message and meaning (e.g, Ruesch & Bateson, 1951). The first involves the actual content of the message and is called the *communication.* The second, called the *metacommunication,* says something about the relationship that is involved between the persons who are interacting. Typically, the communication is conveyed verbally and the metacommunication is conveyed nonverbally. The concept of *double-bind* was developed to describe discrepancies between these two aspects (Bateson et al., 1956).

Double-Bind

A double-bind exists when the discrepancy between the communication and the metacommunication poses a dilemma for the receiver of the conflicting messages. Does the receiver respond to the communication or to the metacommunication? For example, a mother greets her institutionalized son. Verbally she says, "How good it is to see you again." This is the content aspect of her message and is positive in tone. Nonverbally, however, her body stiffens, her hands become rigid, and she holds him at some distance from herself. This is the metacommunicational aspect; it says that she is not eager to be there seeing him. To which message does the boy respond—the positive verbal communication or the rejecting metacommunication? He is said to be caught in a double-bind. If he follows the metacommunication and acts as though she were rejecting, she can counter by claiming she meant what she said verbally; however, if he follows the verbal message, he may respond inappropriately to her real feelings of rejection.

Observers of group interaction can note many instances of the double-bind as well as other discrepancies between communication and metacommunication. They will see, for example, persons verbally communicating one way to their group, while nonverbally expressing an opposing message. The dilemma for the group is to clarify which meaning they should respond to. Senders, of course, may not be aware of their double messages and so will remain puzzled about why people respond to them as they do.

Does Ruth really mean "No, I don't want to take over the leadership" when she utters these words, or do we respond to her metacommunication of apparent eagerness? Does Betty really not want to talk or is she really eager to express her opinions? Suppose someone says to her, "Betty, I've noticed that you have been silent during most of this discussion. Is there anything you would care to tell us about this issue?" She smiles, her eyes brighten noticeably she leans forward in her chair, shuffles her feet, and says, "No, I'm happy just remaining quiet and watching you all discuss the project." Should the questioner then sit back and accept the verbal communication, or decide that she really means what the *metacommunication* reveals—namely that she would like to talk but needs a little more pushing, an invitation to enter into the discussion? If she is taken at her word and isn't pushed a little, she might feel rejected. If she is encouraged to talk, she may provide a useful contribution.

Observers of family interaction often note a similar dilemma, as we see in this example:

> Ralph receives a call at work from Roger, an old family friend. Roger is in town for only one day; without consulting his wife, Ralph invites Roger over for dinner. He then calls up his wife, Sue, to tell her to expect a third for dinner. She says she is eager to see the old family friend, and excitedly prepares the dinner. Later that evening, Ralph and Sue get involved in a rather nasty argument over Roger's coming to dinner. The puzzling fact about their communication is that they are basically in agreement; their argument seems to make little sense. Both agree that it was a great idea to have Roger over for dinner; both were pleased to see him again. But by taking the initiative to invite Roger over for dinner without first consulting his wife, Ralph has declared something about the power relationship between himself and Sue. Their battle is over the power each has in decision-making, a metacommunicational issue. (From Watzlawick, Beavin & Jackson, 1967).

This case is more complex than the simpler double-bind example (e.g., mother and son) or the typical cases involving a discrepancy between what the person says verbally and what she or he says nonverbally (e.g., Ruth or Betty in the group). In this case, we must attend to a complex set of communications between the husband and the wife rather than one or two simple statements. In many different ways, each tells the other how pleased they are to have Roger over, how good it is to see him again, how much they both like him, and so forth. Yet in many different ways, each also implies that it was wrong (from the wife's perspective) or right (from the husband's) for Ralph to have made the decision without consulting Sue. The analysis of this case, therefore, requires a consideration of what are ostensibly paragraphs and pages of interaction rather than a single, isolated message. The point, however, remains the same: there are two discrepant levels of meaning.

In general terms, this case highlights a common aspect of group interaction. People often become involved in heated arguments even while they are in apparent agreement over issues of content. Members may be in apparent agreement over the content of a proposed decision, but cannot actually make and act upon it. They get wrapped up in argumentation and become immobilized. Why? Examine the metacommunicational messages that are involved. These messages often say something about the power and authority relationships that exist and that lead members to resist acting upon decisions that imply, "I have less power than you, because you first suggested the idea."

Hidden Agenda

The metacommunications mentioned above make up much of a group's *hidden agenda*, an agenda that must be adequately dealt with before the group's more formally stated agenda can be satisfactorily negotiated. Recall the discussion in Chapter 8. A hidden agenda is related to socioemotional issues— those that have to do with maintaining internal order and harmony. As we previously noted, unless these matters are resolved, groups will flounder helplessly and ineffectively; the same issues will recur again and again; no decisions or actions will be accomplished, and the group's work will never get done.

The observer can learn to be sensitive to the hidden agendas that are usually conveyed via metacommunication; i.e., to the issues of member-member relationships that are implied even when the members agree about the actual content of their discussion. It is helpful to focus members' attention on their agreements in content in order to clarify for them that the issue lies elsewhere, in their hidden agenda.

"AS-IF" APPROACHES TO ASSESSMENT

To act "as-if " is to take another person's role and attempt to see and experience through his or her eyes. It is by no means an easy thing to do; yet it is an important assessment technique. There are really two related as-if techniques. The first involves the use of actual role-playing within groups in order to better evaluate and understand some aspect of group process. The second asks observers to put themselves figuratively into the situation by empathizing with the persons involved, thereby to gain a better appreciation of what is going on in the group. Let us briefly examine each of these as-if approaches in turn.

Role-Playing

Role-playing techniques can provide a useful approach to understanding. They involve creating a situation that portrays some issue, problem, or event within the group. An example of role-playing will illustrate this point.

> The group contains eight persons, six of whom have been meeting together for several weeks. Two new members will be added to an existing group of six. The leader anticipates that the introduction of the new members will pose an issue that should be dealt with immediately by the group rather than left alone, perhaps to emerge later to interfere with the group's functioning. The leader feels that an issue exists both for the continuing members, who now have to learn about these new people and how to relate to them, and for the two strangers, who must figure out their place in the group. She expects, for example, that the new members will feel isolated from the others, that they may be reluctant to express themselves openly and to participate actively in the group. It is also likely that the continuing members will resent these outsiders and ignore them or put on a show for them: "see how we do things in our group." The leader has decided to confront the new/old issue head on through role-playing. The leader creates a role-playing situation in which an old member portrays a new member and a new member portrays the old. In other words, she creates a *role reversal* so that individuals can gain a better appreciation of the meanings of being "new" and "old" in this group. After the role-playing, a discussion is held in order to explore the feelings and experiences that emerged. Toward the end of the session and at the next meeting, all members express feeling much better about their group than before the role-playing. The new members feel themselves to be an active part of the group; simply having participated in a role-playing exercise has helped integrate them better. Likewise, old members, sensitized to the feelings of being new, are more inclined to incorporate the new persons into their group.

In the example, the leader anticipated an issue and used a role-playing technique, role reversal, to focus attention on this issue and to provide material for group discussion and analysis. In many cases, issues emerge during the course of group interactions that readily lend themselves to some form of role-playing. For example, a conflict between different opinions may be helpfully clarified by asking the participants to role-play the opposing sides, thereby giving everyone a better view of both opinions.

Role-playing need not involve role reversals. The use of role-playing in training proves especially helpful in giving trainees a sense of the kinds of job-related issues they are likely to meet; it gives them and their associates an opportunity to work through these issues in a more concrete way rather than or in addition to discussing them in more general, abstract terms. For example, the nurse who must deal with a dying patient can be helped by role-playing the situation. One person plays the patient while others take on roles as members of the family. The role-playing permits issues to emerge that might not otherwise be confronted except in the real situation. While acting out this situation, the nurse may discover that she tends to avoid talking about the issue with the patient or his family; she may look to the side, avert her gaze, and in other ways communicate her troubles in confronting death. Role-playing allows these aspects of her behavior to come directly to light so they can be dealt with; thus she becomes better prepared to deal with the actual situation when she encounters it.

Role-playing techniques are useful in two aspects of the assessment process: for discovery and for working through issues that have been uncovered. In the example, by role-playing, the nurse is helped to discover her attitudes toward death and dying by seeing these attitudes emerge in her own behavior. In addition to this discovery, role-playing permits her to *work through* her attitudes. She is allowed to try out alternative ways of relating to the patient and his family and to experiment with ways of coping with a potentially difficult situation.

Empathy

The second type of as-if approach involves the process of empathy. Basically, this requires that the observer-practitioner figuratively place him- or herself in the shoes of someone else—this way the individual must ask *"How would I feel if I were that person in these circumstances?"*

A team of health professionals has been meeting to discuss and evaluate the treatment plans for selected cancer patients. An issue emerges between two members who have known one another outside the group and who have formed rather negative feelings that interfere with their functioning within the group. It becomes obvious to everyone that these two may never agree on any proposal that is made because they use all proposals as a vehicle for continuing their outside battle. As a result, the whole group is bogged down and unable to make progress. Thus, it has become imperative to deal with the issue so that the group can function again. But one member of the arguing pair, Janice, refuses to talk about the outside issue. The group leader decides to employ a version of the as-if technique. She figuratively places herself in Janice's shoes, seeking to experience the situation as though she were Janice. The group leader then says, "If I were you, Janice, I would really be angry and upset right now. How do you feel?" This technique, repeated on several different occasions, helps Janice feel that she has an understanding ally; thus she begins to feel free to begin to deal with her own feelings. Soon, the group is able to get back to its major task issues.

In the example, the leader acts as if she *is* the other person and speaks for her, expressing what Janice might feel or want to say but is hesitant to say. Of course, it is possible for the leader to make incorrect assessments or an assessment that is premature and thus is not useful. In this case, the "problem" person will usually simply reject the leader's as-if statements. In the illustration, however, the leader's assessment helped lead the group past this block to its continued progress.

Empathy can be used in groups by either the leader or the members; it can be used in groups of colleagues and of patients. By actively attempting to gain the other person's perspective, to see and to experience the situation from the other side, the health professional is able to make a better assessment of the situation and to intervene in a helpful manner.

Let us examine one further example. A member of the team is dealing with a 44-year-old woman who is facing surgery for breast cancer. By placing herself in that woman's situation, the professional can ask herself: "How would I feel if I were 44, attractive, and facing the possible loss of my breast tomorrow? What kinds of things would I be worried about? I would worry about my husband and how he might feel toward me. I would worry about what else might be found once I was cut open. I would be frightened." Seeing and experiencing from the patient's perspective, as if one is the patient, can be invaluable in the health professional's understanding and intervention.

A Caution

Using oneself as the key assessment tool can involve pitfalls. We too often project ourselves and our own biases onto the other rather than experiencing the situation in that person's terms. The risk, then, is that we might not be acting or experiencing as if we were the other person but rather as we might do or feel. Caution is required. However, in many situations, the feelings are sufficiently common and shared that we can be relatively secure in trying to view the situation through the eyes of another.

OBSERVING VERBAL BEHAVIOR

In observing people's verbal communications, we confront a rich and variable source of material. We can focus on the *content* of what is said, noting, for example, what kinds of questions are asked, what theme or issue are people talking about. And we can focus on the *form* or the ways in which things are expressed—for example, who asks questions and who gives answers? In this latter case, we are not really attending to what is said but rather to its form: that is, it is not the content that we examine, but rather the expression of that content. While it is possible to separate content from form, we are usually interested in observing both features of verbal behavior. Furthermore, we must realize that the content of a verbal communication may be conveyed directly (e.g., "Shut up!"), somewhat indirectly (e.g., "I think it is a bit noisy in here") or very indirectly (e.g., "I went to a film the other night and had great difficulty in hearing, there were so many kids around just talking among themselves"). Let us look at an informative example that illustrates several of these points.

> When the family members gather together with the psychologist and social worker to discuss Mrs. Aberle's pending breast surgery, the psychologist says: "I think it will be helpful if we examine our feelings about the upcoming surgery and use this occasion to ask any questions that you may have." This is what he observes in response:

Observations of Verbal Behavior

1. Mr. Aberle begins to talk about the last time he went to the hospital, noting that it was to the ER for what turned out to be a relatively minor matter.
2. Mrs. Aberle's mother, who lives in the Aberle household, notes that her own health is poor and that she gets anxious whenever she has to go to the hospital: "I just don't trust those doctors."
3. Rob, the 14-year-old son, mentions the cold symptoms he's been having.
4. Gail, the 16-year-old daughter, comments on Rob's never being able to take proper care of himself and how she always has to mother him.
5. Mr. Aberle comments again about his own experiences with doctors and hospitals, noting how things always turn out to be worse in anticipation than in realization.
6. Gwen says to Mr. Aberle, "You just don't understand, do you! I'm frankly worried about it."

The content of much of this family's remarks focuses on each person's experience with illness and with doctors. Mr. Aberle seems to deny that there is really anything to worry about, almost reassuring himself. The patient's mother directly and openly expresses her anxiety about her daughter's operation and expresses the same doubts that her daughter probably also feels. The son, Rob, seems to find it easier to focus on his own problems rather than openly confronting his mother's pending surgery. Gail, in turn, seems to be expressing her anxiety about the new role she will have to take on (mother) as her mother is forced to withdraw from these functions for a while. She might also be expected to be anxious about the implications of breast surgery for herself. The content, therefore, can be very revealing about how each member of this family relates to Mrs. Aberle's surgery and its special meaning to them.

Note that the focus is not simply on the content as such, but on the verbal content as an answer (direct or indirect) to the question, "How do you each feel about the surgery?" Thus, when Mr. Aberle's response is to relate his own recent hospital visit that turned out to be something relatively minor ("I'm not worried—after all it must be minor just like my own experience"), the acute observer will realize that this denial of the seriousness of the procedure is an issue that will have to be dealt with.

The form of the verbal communication in the example above suggests the following: (1) Everyone answers the psychologist's question by personalizing it; that is, all relate one of their own experiences that is intended to carry or convey their feelings in a less direct manner. (2) There is disagreement within the family regarding the seriousness of the surgery. In particular, we note the difference between Mr. Aberle and his mother-in-law. We might even detect some hostility generating between them as she tries to convince everyone of the seriousness of the operation and the problems involved and as he tries to convince everyone that it is not a major matter. (3) All family members except the patient's mother use an indirect mode of expression. She is fairly direct in expressing her concerns.

SOCIOLINGUISTICS

It would take us too far beyond the interests of the introductory level to do more than briefly mention the field of sociolinguistics (Ervin-Tripp, 1969; Gumperz & Hymes, 1972). To oversimplify, the observer uses the structural features of language behavior in order to understand the social relationships that exist within groups. We noted previously, for example, how the forms of address used reflect the degree of formality or informality that is involved within a group as well as the nature of the authority relationship that exists. In a similar manner, the observer can note other features of language and from these learn still more about group processes.

Language Codes

Investigators have demonstrated that most of us are facile in using several different language codes in our everyday conversations (Bernstein, 1971, 1973; Hymes, 1964). For example, we can use a relatively formal code when giving a lecture or speaking in a formal gathering; yet with our friends, we drop some of the formality and switch to more colloquial language forms. Research has shown that by observing just the language code that is used within a group, it is possible to make inferences about the nature of the relationships within that group and about the social status of the members. One investigator (Labov, 1966; 1972) demonstrated the "r-less" quality of street language (e.g., the words, "four," "door," "car" and so forth lose their "r" sound) in New York in contrast to the return of "r" when the same persons are speaking formally or trying to communicate the impression of higher status.

To take another example, one team of investigators (Blom & Gumperz, 1972) noted that when engaged in trading, members of a Norwegian town spoke one language form (standard Norwegian) but switched to another (a local dialect) when dealing with personal matters. That is, they had one language code for business and another for less formal relationships. Clearly, an observer sensitive to these features of language behavior could learn a great deal about a group simply by noting the forms used in communications.

The issue of language code is especially relevant to the health professional in his or her work with patients and with the public (e.g., in community settings, with patient groups, and so forth). It is not unusual, for example,
for medical professionals to communicate in the technical language of their
field and in so doing completely confuse or bypass the patient who is
equipped to understand a far less technical code.

> In a sexuality group, the nurse speaks about coitus, the clitoris, vaginal dis-
> charge, and so forth, assuming that these terms communicate her points to
> the public. The audience leaves without asking questions that might reveal their
> failure to understand and her failure to communicate. They may feel that they
> now have learned something and she may feel that she has taught something.
> And yet no real educational process has occurred.

> In a hospital, the nurse or the nurse's aide is giving the patient a bath.
> She hands the washrag to the patient, saying, "Now you finish your bath—I'll
> be back in a few minutes." When she returns, she notes that the patient has
> washed his hair, his face and his hands, but has not washed the genital area,
> which is what she intended him to do when she left the room. Although her
> language was not technical as such, it was part of a language code that commu-
> nicates only to members of the in-group and not to the patient group for whom
> it is intended.

A sensitivity to and awareness of differences between the language codes
of different groups is essential for the health professional. In these cases,
the codes are not simply informative about the nature of the relationship
that is involved (e.g., whether it involves friends or is more impersonal), but
rather gets to the very heart of professional-patient communication. Professionals must become facile in determining the terms of language usage that
are employed among the patient groups they are working with; they must
then develop a facility in using those codes in order to communicate
and inform.

Language and Thought

Some investigators (Bernstein, 1971; 1973) have proposed the important
hypothesis that language usage and cognitive functioning—that is, the way
people think and respond to one another—are intimately linked. Specifically, it has been suggested that some language codes, termed restricted, make
it difficult to engage in the more subtle aspects of conversation; they constrain people to act more directly and physically rather than using words
to analyze and describe a feeling, a situation, or even a symptom. Some
individuals lack the words and concepts to describe inner bodily events or
to make coherent sense out of things that have happened. Although there
is some evidence that there is a social-class factor at work in these matters—
some class-based language codes make it more difficult and other codes make

it easier to verbally express complex and subtle ideas—more than social class seems to be involved. For the observer of verbal behavior, however, there is a rich territory of material open to systematic observation and analysis.

For the practitioner, of course, these kinds of difference in language codes and ability to provide rich descriptions of symptoms, for example, suggest the importance of developing alternative ways to obtain necessary information from patients. They also suggest that patients may need help in learning the terms and concepts that make the kinds of differentiations that their everyday language does not permit, but which the health professional feels is critical for their practice.

An Example: The Pelvic Exam

Observing how others speak, the forms they use, the manner by which verbal descriptions are generated, what specific terms are employed, can be informative to the trained observer, as is shown in the following example:

> Dr. Joan Emerson (Ph.D.) observed a number of pelvic examinations, noting among other things how the language used by the doctors and the nurses maintained the situation as a medical one rather than as a situation having more directly sexual meanings. She noted, for example, how "medical talk" helped to sustain the setting as nonsexual, whereas the intrusion of nonmedical talk threatened to make the setting inappropriately sexual. The staff used medical terms that help depersonalize the situation; formal terms rather than colloquial terms were used for body parts. Doctors talked about *the* vagina rather than *your* vagina, thereby making it even more impersonal. Instructions to the patient likewise were couched in a language that refuted any possible sexual imagery. Instead of the doctor asking the patient to "spread your legs," with its potential sexual connotations, "Let your knees fall apart" was frequently used. Emerson noted how patients' own language usage sought to minimize the personal quality of the exam; they too referred to pains "down there" or "down below." (From Emerson, 1975)

The trained observer is able to see how the language forms that are used in interaction help shape and sustain the meanings that develop. It is possible to learn a great deal, therefore, by taking careful note of how others express themselves, what address forms they use, what language codes they select, and what terms they employ to describe and to refer to themselves and others.

THE BALES SYSTEM

One of the best-known systems available for systematically analyzing verbal interaction within groups was proposed several years ago by R.F. Bales (1950a;b; 1970). He provides categories that involve the broader aspects of group interaction, encompassing many different kinds of content. Furthermore, although he emphasized the analysis of verbal behavior, he believes the observer should use both verbal and nonverbal cues to make a decision about the category to which a particular utterance should be assigned.

Bales developed his system for observing and recording communication based on his theory regarding the two major areas of concern to all groups: *task issues* and *socioemotional* or *maintenance issues*. We considered these in Chapter 4. Bales reasoned that communication could be primarily concerned with either task matters or maintenance issues. He developed a scheme that distinguished between these two major categories. Communication in the socioemotional or maintenance area, he believed, could be generally positive or generally negative; further, a distinction could be made within the task area as well. Bales therefore sought to distinguish between communications that *give out* material to others and those that *ask for* material from others. With these several distinctions in mind, Bales developed a twelve-category system for observing and recording communication within groups.

I. Communication Involving Task Issues

A. Giving or Sending to Others

1. Gives Suggestion: involves taking some lead and direction in task matters, including focusing the group's attention on a problem, organizing the group, developing an agenda, and so forth.

2. Gives Opinion: involves serious evaluation and analysis or commentary on the task, including reasoning, judgment, elaboration, diagnosis, etc.

3. Gives Orientation: involves providing information and clarification of points and issues, helping to orient the group to its task, conveying knowledge relevant to dealing with the task.

B. Asking for or Receiving Material From Others

4. Asks for Suggestion: involves a concern that is parallel to category #1; emphasizes needing some direction, requesting an agenda, turning the initiative over to another, etc.

5. Asks for Opinion: parallels category #2; seeks to elicit or to encourage reactions on the part of others; tries to elicit opinions from others on various items and issues that come before the group.

6. Asks for Orientation: parallels category #3; involves seeking factual type information or clarification of still confusing matters.

II. Communications Involving Maintenance Issues

A. Emotionally Positive Expressions

7. Shows Solidarity: involves acting in a generally supportive and friendly way, helpful to others, caring of others, expressing harmony and unity.

8. Shows Tension Release: involves acts that joke, laugh, or dramatize in such a way as to help break tension or produce a sense of elation.

9. Agrees: involves acceptance, concurrence, compliance with others, understanding others, being receptive and interested.

B. Emotionally Negative Expressions

10. Disagrees: withholds help from others; passively rejects others; can also include showing disbelief in others' comments or ideas; non-responsive.

11. Shows Tension: symptoms of anxiety and tension, including inappropriate laughter, excessive hesitation, tremor, blocking in speech; may also involve withdrawal and hanging back from issues; showing fear or apprehension.

12. Shows Antagonism: involves unfriendly acts, acts that deflate others, that are defensive, that seem presumptuous or condescending; also includes acts that indicate alienation from others, boredom, noncaring, lack of concern.

To use Bales's system, we should not only learn the meaning of each category; we also must learn to record communications on a who-to-whom matrix over time. Thus, to use this scheme in a systematic manner, we would indicate:

—WHO: which group member is speaking?

—SAYS WHAT: into which of the twelve categories is the utterance to be located?

—TO WHOM: which member receives the message, or is it directed to the group in general?

—WHEN: when in the sequence of the meeting is the comment made?

Uses

Admittedly, it is likely that only a researcher interested in obtaining a complete record of a group's communication patterns would use the Bales method in the manner indicated. The results of such work, however, can be rather striking. They would reveal a literal structure to the communication within a group, an outline of who contributes the most to group task and maintenance functions—e.g., who, though speaking a great deal, seems to contribute little; who is relatively antagonistic; who responds to whom; and so on. The time-sequencing analysis permits the investigator to discover developmental trends in the life of the group.

If it is primarily the researcher who will use a scheme such as that of Bales in the systematic manner he suggests, then what use is such an approach to the health professional who simply wants to evaluate the status of a group? In our view, even though one might not use the Bales system (or some similar system) in precisely the way proposed, it does provide a way of systematically observing and thinking about interaction and communication within groups. It has been our experience that those who train themselves to use these categories become better observers of group interaction. They become sensitized to aspects of communication that the more casual observer tends to overlook. Thus, even though we might not be as systematic or complete as the researcher in our use of Bales system, efforts to practice observing interaction with this system will help increase our sensitivity to and awareness of communication within a group.

SUMMARY AND CONCLUSIONS

A convenient way of summarizing the complex interrelationship of verbal and nonverbal materials that are used in the assessment of group and individual process is represented in Table 11-1. This table provides a model that organizes the material introduced in this chapter (and several other chapters we have considered e.g., chapters on theory) so that it can be used for purposes of assessment.

Several case examples using the material summarized in this chapter, as presented in Table 11-1, are presented for the reader's convenience in applying the principles of the assessment process.

Table 11-1. The Assessment Process

I. Perception:	What do I see?	Attention to nonverbal behaviors
	What do I hear?	Attention to nonverbal and verbal behaviors
II. Affect-Empathy:	How do I feel?	Attention to empathy; place self in the other's situation in order to better appreciate

and understand his/her concerns

III. Cognition:	What does it mean?	Development of hunches and tentative interpretations of the meaning of the observed behaviors; includes the on-going examination of additional material that confirms or refutes hunches
IV. Validation:	Is my assessment correct?	Involves testing the assessment: e.g., by asking questions; waiting to gather additional material; checking with others' assessments
V. Intervention:	How shall I respond?	Involves making a decision based on the assessment regarding what actions to take: e.g., to intervene in a supportive way; to probe and question further, etc.

Case #1

The patient, Mrs. Percell, is a 44-year-old woman who has been hospitalized for a breast biopsy. You are talking with her before the full procedure. You are aware that she has had several previous contacts with medical personnel and so is assumed to be relatively well-informed about what will take place and its implications.

Perception

You see Mrs. Percell sitting across from you, clenching her hands, rubbing them together frequently. She appears restless and moves about in her chair. She seems unable to sit still. Her legs, in particular, move. Her face muscles, especially around her lips, are tightened. Her speech is rapid; vocal pitch is high. Occasionally her voice cracks, at which moments she laughs nervously and then covers her mouth with her fingers. The content of her talk involves questions about her pending surgical procedure. This procedure has already been explained to her several times, yet she continues to focus her questions around its details. You notice that she frequently repeats the same question even after you have given what you think is a satisfactory answer.

Affect-Empathy

Ask yourself how you would feel in her situation: you are 44, still young and fairly attractive. You know that you are awaiting a procedure that might result in the loss of one breast; you also know that even more than that can be involved. Frankly, you are frightened and worried about how you will look afterwards and who you will be to your husband, children, friends.

Cognition

You can interpret the various observations as meaning that Mrs. Percell is anxious and is concerned about several issues pertaining to the impact of the procedure on her life. You can sense that these are the real matters that she needs to discuss with someone rather than the minor details that most of her questions seem to center on.

Validation

You directly ask Mrs. Percell if she would find it helpful to talk over with you some of the implications of the biopsy for her and her life.

Intervention

In part, your effort to validate your interpretation is the first step in intervention. You are not only asking her to check out and validate or refute your interpretation; in asking, you are indicating to her that you are sensitive to, aware of, and concerned about her feelings at this time. You are really inviting her to talk things over with you. You can then continue your intervention by suggesting, for example, that it must be a very frightening experience and that she might like to discuss that aspect with you. You could inquire about her husband: Has she talked things over with him yet? What was his reaction? How does she feel about his response to her? What concerns does she have about him? What other concerns and worries does she have?

Case #2

You are dealing with male post-coronary patients whose group you organized to help discuss and deal with issues of daily living. They eagerly signed up to attend several workshops under your direction; you assumed that their eagerness was motivated by their many questions and concerns that had not been resolved by other medical personnel with whom they had had contact.

Perception

You note that several of the men are restless, moving about in their chairs. Several look up toward the ceiling; a few gaze intently out the window. One or two open their mouth and take in a deep breath as though they are preparing to speak, but then say nothing. There are frequent silences, broken on occasion by desultory conversation. The voice quality of those who speak is very soft and hesitant. You are impressed by their tendency almost to speak in a whisper as if to save energy and avoid strain. The content of their talk tends to wander about; there are a few jokes made about sports and an occasional hint about something vaguely sexual. A couple briefly mention their jobs; and one member mentions something about being a man, but this is quickly dropped, replaced by a joke—and then silence.

Affect-Empathy

You realize that most of these men are in their late 40s to early 50s. They still have family concerns, children in college to support, large mortgage payments, jobs that are threatened by a tight job market. Place yourself in their situation and ask how you would feel if you were in their position. What kinds of concerns would you have? You would feel anxious about being able to function as you did before. Could you really keep your job and support your family? And if you couldn't, then what kind of a man would you be? And what about your sex life? Can you continue as before or must that too come to an end? And if you can't keep a job and can't keep active sexually, then who are you? Is life still worth living?

Cognition

You would interpret the various indicators as suggesting that most of the members of the group are anxious, but perhaps not yet clear about just what all their concerns are. Perhaps they are even a bit embarrassed about mentioning what they might consider to be private and personal matters of jobs and sex, and so they engage in rather indirect and desultory conversation.

Validation

Check your interpretation by saying something such as the following to the entire group: "I've noticed that we seem to have trouble getting started, trouble in talking about what some of our real concerns are. I wonder if people here are somewhat embarrassed to talk about what most worries them now? I realize that it may be difficult, but I wonder—are people here anxious about the effects of their coronary on their ability to continue their job, to continue maintaining a family, to continue their usual sexual activities? Maybe these are some of the things we should try and talk about."

Intervention

In validating your hunch, you have already begun to intervene in the process of this group. It is important from this point on that you as a health professional be continually attentive to specific persons in the group and their modes of expression so that you can make it easy for each member to air his concerns and share with others.

12

Leadership Issues, Types, and Approaches

"Leaders are born, not made." "Either you have what it takes to be a leader or you don't; there's no in between." "He's good at taking orders, but I'd never want him to lead the group." "She's a natural leader; there's nothing more she needs to learn about leadership." "Hell, it makes no difference who you're leading—they all need the same strong direction." "My best groups are those in which I don't do anything; they take the lead and it works fine."

*L*eadership has fascinated people since the beginnings of society. Who shall lead and who shall follow has often been of greater importance than where shall we go. Aristotle subscribed to the "great man" theory contained in several of our opening statements: that leaders are born, not made. Early studies located leadership in the personality of the leader. Numerous investigations were designed to determine those critical traits of personality and character that would help identify the leader (Bass, 1960; Stogdill, 1948 for summaries). Not surprisingly, a substantial list of traits did emerge, but so too did several important counter-examples:

Leaders tend to be bigger and heavier than followers (Adolph Hitler?); stronger and healthier (Julius Caesar?); handsome and physically more attractive (Abraham Lincoln?); more aggressive and domineering (Mohandas Gandhi?); psychologically well adjusted (Nero?); more intelligent (please provide your own counter-example). In 1972 a political pundit pointed out that Americans prefer taller persons as president and that in every presidential election up until that time the taller of the two candidates had been elected. He predicted therefore, that George McGovern would handily defeat Richard Nixon. (Raven & Rubin, 1976, p. 372)

It may be, then, that leaders are made and not born.

LEADERSHIP AND THE SITUATION

As we think more critically about leadership, even our common sense directs us toward several different factors that go into leadership: personality and character, situation, task, and members. When the situation, members, and type of task are held fairly constant, certain personality traits emerge to describe group leaders. For example, dominance and assertiveness have been found to characterize the leaders of all-male groups in military-type contexts performing fairly routine problem-solving tasks. A change in personnel, setting, or task, however, reveals a different set of leadership traits. The person who can lead one type of group facing one type of task may not be the best to lead a different group facing a different task, e.g., Nurse Armstrong may be good in leading a group composed primarily of other nurses discussing a treatment plan, but may not be capable of leading a group of various other health professionals engaged in developing a proposal for a community-wide health-care program.

WHAT IS MEANT BY LEADERSHIP?

To what are we referring when we talk about "leadership" and "leaders?" There are several possibilities (Gibb, 1969):

1. One person who has been assigned the office or position of leader. This is often referred to as *headship* in order to distinguish between the formally appointed group leader and persons who informally take on group leadership.
2. Several persons who serve leadership functions, who act in those ways necessary for the group to work effectively toward its goals.
3. A person who is the central focus for the group, around whom the group forms and whose presence is necessary for the group's continuation and cohesiveness.
4. A person who is the most influential, who has the most power or the greatest ability to affect and alter the behavior of others.

Each of these describes an aspect of leadership. It is generally agreed that the most fruitful approach to the study of leadership is one that focuses on leadership functions rather than on a specific person as such (Cartwright & Zander, 1968; Gibb, 1969). The questions of leadership are thereby directed toward understanding the nature of these functions and their distribution within a group: e.g., does one person always serve a particular function or is there a more equal distribution of functions across the membership? By focusing our attention on leadership functions, we also increase our sensitivity to the kinds of skills and knowledge that *all* people are able to bring to the group. Many individuals can and do serve leadership functions even though they may not have been formally appointed to such a position or have the title of group leader. Thus, by considering leadership as referring to *functions* rather than to persons, we can examine who serves those functions and how those functions are served within any particular group. We will note that at times the formally appointed group leader will serve many of the necessary functions; however, we will also note those times at which members come forward and serve necessary leadership functions.

Leadership Functions

What is meant by "leadership functions?" The list of leadership functions is extensive but usually includes the following (Lippitt, 1961):

1. Helping the group decide on its purposes and goals.
2. Helping the group focus on its own process of working together so that it may become more effective rather than becoming trapped by faulty ways of problem-solving and decision-making.
3. Helping the group become aware of its own resources and how best to use them.
4. Helping the group evaluate its progress and development.
5. Helping the group to be open to new and different ideas without becoming immobilized by conflict.
6. Helping the group learn from its failures and frustrations as well as from its successes.

In talking about leadership functions, we are talking about actions and behaviors that any group member may carry out. Successful groups require that these functions be dealt with. No one person, however, need handle all of them. In fact, it is unlikely that a single person will be capable of effectively handling the multiplicity of functions that are necessary for the group to work well. Therefore, function #3 becomes important in most groups. The designated leader must work to utilize the resources and abilities of other members in order to handle the functions that he or she cannot personally manage.

Effective Leadership

Our analysis suggests that when we talk about leadership we are really referring to leadership functions. In this view, the skills of leadership involve the ability to get others to participate in leadership functions rather than in taking on the entire burden oneself. Leadership involves the effective utilization of a group's total resources; although one person may be designated group leader, effective resource utilization means that all members serve important leadership functions.

LEADERSHIP AS THE FACILITATION OF ASSETS OVER LIABILITIES

When a group comes together to work on a task or solve a problem, there are certain potential *assets* and certain potential *liabilities* that can develop (Maier, 1970). Let us briefly review some of these potential assets and liabilities.

ASSET: Since a group is composed of several individuals, there is often a wide and diverse range of ideas and information that can be called upon to solve a problem, make a decision, or get a job completed.

LIABILITY: Even though diversity exists, there are social pressures in all groups; members want to be accepted by others in their group. Often, the price of this acceptance is the avoidance of disagreements. Thus, diversity is silenced as members hope to gain acceptance by concealing rather than expressing their differences.

ASSET: Most solutions to issues and problems require their acceptance by members before they can be implemented. When members participate actively in their group, they are likely to accept the decisions that have been made. Furthermore, because decisions must be communicated from the decision-makers to those who will implement them, the involvement of the latter with the former can help minimize distortion and faulty communication.

LIABILITY: Not everyone participates equally in the work of a group. Dominant members or a dominant leader may persuade others to adopt a solution that they really do not accept or agree with. Thus, when it comes time for them to implement the decision, they drag their feet or do it poorly. Furthermore, communications among members within a group can be distorted as members try to gain personal acceptance from others, to look good, and so forth.

Now that we have a sense of some of the possible assets and liabilities that stem from group work, let us examine the way in which a leader can influence whether a particular item will be an asset or a liability.

Diversity

The diversity of opinion, fact, and perspective that characterizes groups can be an asset if this diversity is brought to bear on problem-solving; it can be a liability, however, if conflict and hard feelings develop among group members. A leader can try to reduce the expression of the diversity among members and thereby minimize conflict; yet the cost of doing this is to minimize the full utilization of the resources that diversity offers. And so, a leader can try to implement disagreement.

Certain leadership behaviors are helpful in creating a climate within which disagreement can be generated without running the risk of hard feelings and excessive, destructive conflict (Maier, 1970):

1. The leader is open to perceiving disagreements rather than denying their presence.

2. The leader adopts a permissive attitude, one that allows members to express diverse opinions without fear of ridicule or rejection.

3. The leader helps the group to delay rushing into a decision so that a fuller discussion can be generated and disagreements explored.

4. The leader helps the group to process its diverse information and perspectives.

5. The leader structures sessions so that a period of idea generation is separated from a period of idea evaluation.

6. The leader structures sessions so as to keep the group focused on its issues and its goals and not lost in conflict or side issues.

7. The leader helps the group focus on its mutual interests rather than emphasizing conflict; the leader helps the group realize that its mutual interests can be served through the open expression of disagreement as long as the long-range goals are kept clearly in mind.

8. The leader helps those with minority or unpopular opinions to express them; the leader acts in ways to protect dissenters from harassment, ridicule, or rejection.

A Conclusion

Although any member can serve leadership functions, the designated leader or organizer bears a special responsibility to help a group use its resources as assets rather than as liabilities. A review of the listed leader behaviors that help a characteristic such as diversity become an asset rather than a liability suggests the importance of the leader's attitude, philosophy, and style. Basically, a person's style of leadership affects whether a particular characteristic of a group will become an asset or a liability. This suggests that it is important to understand the concept of leadership *style*.

LEADERSHIP STYLE

When we talk about a style of leadership, we are simply referring to the typical ways in which a person takes on the leadership role within a group. Leadership style can be seen to be a result of the person's underlying theory of human nature. Leadership style, in turn, results in a particular set of consequences for the group that is being led. We can organize our thinking about leadership style through the following diagram:

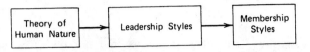

Figure 12-1. Antecedents and outcomes of leadership style.

The diagram indicates that the theory of human nature a person maintains will influence the particular style of group leadership he or she adopts. That style, in turn, will influence the ways in which the members of the group behave together. To more fully appreciate this diagram and its implications, we must begin our inquiry with an examination of some underlying theories of human nature that are related to leadership styles.

Theories of Human Nature

Several years ago, McGregor (1960) introduced the idea that people varied in their conception of human nature. He spoke of Theory X and Theory Y conceptions. The Theory X person, according to McGregor, believes that other people:

1. Dislike work and so avoid it if they can,
2. Must be coerced, controlled, and even threatened into working, and
3. Have little ambition or stomach for responsibility and so really enjoy being directed and strongly led.

The Theory Y person believes that:

1. Effort expended in work is as natural and pleasurable as effort expended in play,
2. People are capable of exercising self-direction and self-control once they feel committed to certain objectives and goals, and
3. People not only learn to accept but actively seek areas in which they can be autonomous and responsible.

The implication of this theory of leadership practice is fairly self-evident. People subscribing to Theory X would be likely to engage in what Maier (1970) terms a leadership style of "persuasive selling." They would believe it essential to direct and to control others. They would not trust others to be responsible or to be able to take any initiative and would see their own role therefore as demanding a high level of control, dominance, and supervision. Theory Y leaders, by contrast, would be more likely to engage in a "problem-solving" style of leadership. Basically, their goal would focus on helping the group solve problems rather than on accepting the leaders' own pre-formed opinion.

Self-Fulfilling Prophecy

An intriguing quality of these philosophies and their associated styles of group leadership is their self-fulfilling nature. That is, it is not surprising to find that group members led by Theory X leaders require direction and close supervision; they seem to lack initiative and appear unable to do things on their own without the leader's presence and guidance. The leader's theory about human nature is thereby validated by the group's behavior. That this leader's own style of leadership may have contributed to this style of membership often escapes notice. There is good reason to believe, however, that a particular leadership style gives rise to a particular membership style; the latter is usually one that confirms the leader's ideas about human nature and thus a prophecy is fulfilled and a leadership style justified.

The Democratic, Autocratic, and Laissez-Faire Leadership Styles

One of the best known descriptions of leadership style was formulated some years ago by Lewin, Lippitt, and White (Lippitt & White, 1958). It differentiates between a member-centered problem-solving style termed *democratic*, a leader-centered "persuasive selling" style termed *autocratic*, and a noncentered style termed *laissez-faire*.

Democratic Leadership Style

This member-centered leadership style tends to follow from the Theory Y concept of human nature; it emphasizes the utilization of the resources within groups that are available and must be tapped. Its design is to create a climate within which members can openly express themselves, share their diversity without fear of rejection or excessive conflict, explore their different skills and talents, and build upon these in accomplishing their mutual tasks. Democratic leaders adopt a problem-solving perspective; their goal is to help members achieve their own ends rather than sell the group the leaders' views or ideas.

The democratic style is very active; its mission basically is to facilitate the members' participation in decisions, formulating and evaluating policy, considering alternatives, taking action. The leader's efforts are directed toward including all members in the groups activities and decisions. Some specific aspects of this style include the following:

1. The leader works with the members in developing plans that are agreeable to everyone rather than telling members exactly what they are to do and how they are to do it.

2. The leader's statements are intended to guide rather than to direct.

3. The leader takes on responsibility for helping the group evaluate its progress; also intervenes to help the group keep to its agenda and not stray too far from its goals.

4. The leader gives expert information only when it is pertinent to the situation at hand; he or she does not use expertise irrelevantly to gain status.

5. The leader supports spontaneous shifts in direction and the methods that emerge from within the group that all agree are within the limits defined by the group. (from Deutsch, Pepitone & Zander, 1948)

Autocratic Leadership Style

The autocratic style is leader-centered rather than member-centered. Autocratic leaders feel that they know best; their main task is conceived as convincing others of the correctness of their own views: they engage in "persuasive selling." They stifle disagreement within the group unless it helps them better achieve their own personal ends (a divide-and-conquer strategy). They tend to be secretive in their dealings with members, believing that members should be prevented from knowing too much. Keeping group members in the dark about what the goals are and what the relation is between present activities and these goals is a typical technique of autocratic leaders. Such people are proficient at covering over issues that might thwart achievement of their own ends for the group. The group, for them, is not a locus of human resources that need to be tapped but a means of accomplishing personal goals.

The autocratic style need not be nor typically is a hostile or aggressive style (Bradford & Lippitt, 1961). Such leaders can be very personable, even warm and friendly. However, their essential message to the members says, "Let me handle it, I know best." Hard-boiled autocrats seek to secure discipline and conformity to their directive without questioning; the more benevolent autocrat appears to be interested in group members and appears to work closely with them (a pat on the back, a friendly smile of reassurance). The autocratic message remains much the same: "You did it my way and I'm pleased." The autocrat tends to foster excessive dependency on his or her way; they are the groups central focus, and without them no action can be taken, no decisions made.

A frequent variant on the autocratic style is found among people who use what appears to be a democratic, member-centered approach but only as a more complex and sophisticated method for covering over their own persuasive purposes. These people may appear to court member opinion and appear to be open to listening, but only in the name of being a better salesperson; their true interests are in reality to convince the group about their views rather than to help the members develop and express and work with their own resources.

An Example

While the following example (which we first introduced in Chapter 10) combines both the democratic and autocratic styles, it particularly demonstrates how a leader may give the appearance of advocating member participation, yet be involved in manipulating the group to adopt a policy that had already been determined.

The hospital administration, without consulting either the Director of Nursing or the nursing staff, had decided, entirely on the basis of its budgetary concerns, to increase the use of nursing aides on all nursing services at the hospital. This decision was made autocratically, wherein members of the groups most immediately affected by the decision were given no opportunity to be involved in the process of its making. The administration then informed the Director of Nursing of its decision and asked her to present this to the entire nursing staff. Again, an autocratic process was in effect: The Director was told what she was to do and was at no time involved in the decision process.

At this point, an interesting transformation occurred. The Director, rather than passing the message down to her staff—simply continuing the autocratic and hierarchical mode of leadership that was in effect—decided to act as though her nursing staff still had a choice and invited them to participate in a decision process. As you may recall from our previous presentation of this example, she asked her nursing staff to consider the feasibility of using individuals other than R.N.s to provide quality nursing care. Because the decision to use non-R.N.s had already been made, asking them to consider whether or not this use was feasible was effectively involving them in a pseudo-participation. Ultimately, when her nursing staff came back from several weeks of meetings to tell the Director that they had concluded that using non-R.N.s was not feasible, she had to act autocratically and reject their suggestion. This, naturally, created a great deal of anger among her staff and deep distrust of her motives and leadership style.

At this point, the administration intervened. They informed the nurses that although the basic decision to use nursing aides had been made, the manner by which they would be used would be left entirely up to the nursing staff and that furthermore, each floor could develop its own unique plan for such utilization. In other words, one part of the decision had been made autocratically and without their participation, while another part was left entirely open for their full participation and, indeed, determination. Each floor met several times and developed its own manner of utilizing nursing aides. The nursing staff came away from this experience with positive feelings about the honesty of the administration in dealing with them on this matter but continued to feel anger and distrust over the duplicity employed by the Director of Nursing. Finally, they felt good about the plans they had each developed.

It seems clear from this example that an autocratic style, not presented in an arrogant or hostile manner, can work effectively when persons are not going to have any input into a decision. It also seems clear that attempting to simulate democratic leadership, when the facts are otherwise, undermines the leader's rapport with the group and makes it highly unlikely that future leadership from this person will work effectively. Finally, it is also clear that a democratic style that provides people with full participation works very well when it is real; that is, when the decisions reached by the group will be implemented and not overturned because they displease the leader.

Laissez-Faire Leadership Style

This third type of leadership style is neither member- nor leader-centered; rather, it is almost a noncentered style. As the French word suggests, its essence is simply to let things alone to develop as they will. Laissez-faire leaders tend to be a bit withdrawn from any active involvement in the group; they take non-directiveness to its extreme. They do not seek to engage members in discussions, or to facilitate member involvement and participation; nor do they take the total burden into their own hands. They sit back and act as though everything will eventually work out. This style is characterized by the tendency simply to let things drift; clear goals for the group are never formulated; decisions are not made; ongoing evaluation of group process is missing.

This is a style that one sees increasingly among those who have come to distrust all forms of authority and who seem to feel that the best type of leader is the nonleader. Unfortunately, the results of such a style tend to be confusion and nonfunctioning. Or members' frustration builds and they turn to an autocratic member of the group to provide them directive leadership.

Ms. Brady, a nursing instructor, was the group leader for fifteen baccalaureate students in their first term. These students began with no idea of nursing process. At her supervisory sessions, Ms. Brady reported that her group was so relaxed and so together that they really did not need any type of leadership or direction from her. She just let them do anything they wanted: "Today, for example, I sat back and read a newspaper while two students studied for a meds exam, three wandered in and out over the two-hour session, and some others talked. It was really great." Her idea of leadership was to let the group do whatever they wanted. The group never became a cohesive unit; they never really talked together about nursing or about much of anything. They learned nothing.

THE RESULTS OF DIFFERENT STYLES: FROM LEADERSHIP STYLE TO MEMBERSHIP STYLE

We have painted a picture of the various styles of leadership in rather broad strokes, leaving aside the many individual variations that are possible. We can also paint an equally general picture of some of the major consequences that derive from each of the styles. These have been alluded to in several examples. What is important to realize is the degree to which a particular leadership style *produces* a corresponding membership style, even one that all parties may agree is not desirable.

Following is a summary of the membership styles that derive from the three major types of leadership behavior.

Democratic Membership Style

1. Members display a high degree of enthusiasm for their work and considerable involvement and commitment to their work and to their group.

2. A high degree and quality of productivity is generated, giving members the added satisfaction of having participated significantly in producing something of high quality.

3. There is a high degree of group cohesiveness, sense of comradeship, and good morale.

4. Members learn to take on personal responsibilities and to take the initiative; they are able to work effectively even when the leader is late or absent. In the original Lippitt and White research, for example, members continued working when the leader had to leave the room; likewise, they began working even when the leader arrived late. This behavior indicated their general independence from the leader and their ability to take on individual responsibility and initiative for themselves.

5. Members begin to learn leadership skills and effective leader behavior.

6. There is a high degree of motivation and participation. There are few, if any, apathetic members.

Autocratic Membership Style

1. There is much resentment and bitterness over having submitted to the leader. There may be incipient revolts that only the presence of the leader can contain. This has been described by Lippitt and White as a pot ready to boil over; only the leader's presence can keep the lid on.

2. No one takes on any personal responsibility or shows any initiative; there is much buck-passing and resistance to the work. Lippitt and White's data indicate, for example, that members of autocratically led groups do not begin work or continue work without the presence of the leader to spur them on.

3. Symptoms of irritability and resentment show up increasingly: lateness; petty anger over minor matters; apathy. Lippitt and White's data indicate how members scapegoat one another or scapegoat an outsider who comes into the room while the leader is absent. The scapegoat is used as the target for the anger members fear to express directly toward the leader.

4. Productivity may be high, but constant surveillance and supervision are required to maintain it. Turnover may be substantial, resulting in long-term reduction of productive efficiency.

5. Members fail to learn how to function independently, thus few new ideas or innovations develop.

6. Group morale and cohesiveness are low.

Laissez-Faire Membership Style

1. There is low member morale and minimal interest in the task or in the group.

2. There is low group cohesiveness and minimal member concern for one another.

3. Work tends to be sloppy and inefficient; productivity is low.

4. Irritability and unrest tend to be general and unfocused, often building around a feeling of confusion and frustration about the group's drift and inability to get off the ground.

5. There may be much scapegoating as members search around for someone or something to blame for their frustrations.

6. Members are not trained in any leadership skills. They tend to withdraw from active involvement; they become apathetic and bored.

SOME OBJECTIONS TO THE
DEMOCRATIC STYLE

There are some who object to the democratic, member-centered style. It sounds good in theory, critics say, but has little place in practice. In particular, some feel that medical and nursing practice are founded on a hierarchy of expertise in which member participation can only weaken the expert's proper role and result in poor work. In this section we will examine three related answers to these objections concerning the democratic leadership style. The first examines the need for *flexibility* in leadership style; the second investigates the difficulties involved when one person tries to take on *opposing styles* of leadership; the third looks at the effects of leadership style on the *acceptance* of decisions.

Flexibility

When To Be More Directive

There are settings and circumstances in which a clearly defined line of authority is necessary; in which one decision-maker must integrate information, decide, and get others to follow his or her directives. Some research (e.g., Fiedler, 1967) has suggested the importance of a more autocratic leadership style when tasks are highly structured, when the leader has substantial member support and acceptance for his or her ideas, or when the group's situation is such that without strong direction it will fall apart.

For example, on a highly structured task, one in which the alternatives are limited (in the extreme, there may be only one choice to make), a more directive approach may be warranted. Excessive member involvement in the decision process would only serve to delay the inevitable or so confuse members that their cooperation is actually less than it would have been with a more directive leader. However, when the task has many alternatives, when much information is needed, when issues of value and ethics are involved, the more democratic approach is warranted. This would seem to be the case in much work within the health professions: different points of view regarding patient management exist; no single clear solution is present; information from several different sources (e.g., medical, nursing, social workers, etc.) is needed for proper patient care.

The Issue of Rigidity

The problem, of course, is that most persons who engage in leadership functions tend to rigidly adhere either to one style or the other, thereby disregarding the unique characteristics of the situation and the task. In this case, one may be either rigidly democratic or rigidly autocratic in style, rather than adopting an approach that fits the special circumstances that are involved. Typically, however, it is rigid adherence to a Theory X, autocratic style that dominates even in situations and with tasks for which this is not essential and may even be detrimental. It is less typical to find persons behaving in rigidly democratic ways even on tasks in which only one solution is possible.

The skills that are required for democratic leadership are much more demanding and complex than those required for the other styles. In the case of autocratic leadership, one must have a good sense of his or her own position and then work to persuade others or demand that others adopt it. In the democratic style, however, a person must basically work with group process: i.e., adopt the problem-solving perspective and be oriented toward the utilization of members as resources for group action.

The democratic style demands that leaders be willing to reorient their own ideas so that they are no longer concerned with personally winning, or not losing, a point. In the name of winning, many a leader or member has turned to the autocratic style. If it is important for me to have my ideas recognized as originating with me, if it is important for me to be able to say at the conclusion of the meeting that the group has adopted my plat-form and done what I suggested, then I am not likely to be able to do more than try to steer the group along the lines I wish for them. But if I can accept neither winning nor losing—that is, if I can agree that the process of mem-ber involvement in discussion and decision is more important than my own ideas—then I can begin to act in ways that help members explore, examine, and evaluate their own points of view and suggestions.

Assuming Opposing Leadership Styles

Several years ago, Bales (we previously considered some of his works) suggested that we are not likely to find what he termed a "great-man" leader (Bales, 1955; 1958; Borgatta, et al., 1954). By this he meant that few people have the capabilities of simultaneously serving what he termed the task func-tions and the socioemotional functions of the group. Task functions have to do with getting the work done; they may require a leader to be directive or at least to focus on what are at times the less pleasant aspects of accom-plishing goals. Socioemotional functions have to do with the human rela-tions side of group work, with emphasis on group harmony and cohesiveness. It was Bale's contention, based both on theory and his research, that only rarely can one and the same person press a group on to do its tasks and simultaneously help group members deal with interpersonal issues.

One way of thinking about this difficulty is to assume that effective work on the group's task usually necessitates some division of labor: individuals take on different aspects of the total job that has to be done. These differ-ences, in turn, highlight the distinctions between the members. A kind of status hierarchy tends to emerge, and with it invidious comparisons, compe-tition, and jealousy. Socioemotional issues, on the other hand, tend to involve ways in which members are similar—things they share in common (e.g., equal-ity of pay, of respect, of status).

Bales suggested that it is very difficult for one person to push members toward inequality on the one hand (by focusing on task issues) and at the same time push them toward equality (by focusing on socioemotional issues). Hence, no "great-person" leader—no one person who can serve both sets of functions for the group. As we have already noted, the autocratic style may indeed get members to work on their tasks; yet in its failure to deal with interpersonal issues, this method may create tensions and resent-ments that in the long run thwart group effectiveness. But what about a more democratic style?

Feedback Ratio

As part of one of his investigations, Bales (1958) developed the concept of the *feedback ratio*. This was conceived as a measure of the degree to which a person who sends out considerable communication to others (e.g., talks a great deal and seems to dominate) allows communication back from others. A high feedback ratio indicates that there is a reasonable proportionality between what is sent out and what is allowed back in return. A low ratio, by contrast, indicates that someone sends out much, but allows little back. Bales posited that persons with a high feedback ratio were more likely to be "great-person" leaders than those with low ratios. In other words, the leader who courts considerable participation from members is more likely to satisfy both task and socioemotional demands. This, of course, is descriptive of the democratic, member-centered leadership style.

The leader with a low feedback ratio does not approximate the "great-person" leader; he or she tends to dominate a discussion, contributing much to task issues while failing to consider socioemotional functions. In that both sets of functions must be dealt with for a group to work together effectively in the long run, leaders with a low feed-back ratio are not helpful. In fact, they contribute to socioemotional conflicts by their domination. This, of course, is one of the outcomes of the more autocratic style.

The Issue of Acceptance

Maier (1970) points out what initially appears to be a paradox, one that seems especially at issue in the health professions. Leaders often feel that they hold the key to high-quality solutions to the problems and issues within the groups they lead. They sense that they really do know what is best by virtue of their training, experience, and expertise. As they may experience it, the only problem is how to get others to accept their expertise. The paradox arises when the issue of acceptance is analyzed. Here it is important to note first that more decisions are ineffective because they lack the acceptance of those who must adopt and implement them than because they lack quality. Second, acceptance may best be gained if the efforts to sell one's expertise to others is abandoned and those others are brought into more equal partnership: i.e., via a democratic leadership style.

The issue of leadership cannot be divorced from the issue of acceptance. It does us little good to hold all the expertise and wisdom in the world if others do not accept the fruits of this wisdom. Health professionals may fervently believe in their own correctness and expertise and be unable to understand why their patients may fail to heed their advice except when under direct surveillance (e.g. they take their medications when we watch them, but not on their own).

TECHNIQUES OF GROUP LEADERSHIP: PROCESSING AND FEEDBACK

A review of the functions of leadership suggests the following to be important elements:

—Obtaining and receiving information

—Helping in the diagnosis of group goals, obstacles, and consequences of decision choices

—Facilitating communication

—Helping integrate the various perspectives and alternative possibilities for policy or action that emerge within the group

—Testing and evaluating proposals and decisions

Although these are separable aspects of leadership, more significantly, they all require skills in what we will term *processing*.

The Processing Functions of Leadership

Processing requires rather complex perceptual and cognitive abilities in addition to the interpersonal skills it also demands from the group's leader. When we process interactions we focus on the immediate situation that is present here and now. This requires an ability to be at some distance from the immediate, ongoing situation even while actively participating in it. Distance provides the perspective on the immediate present that is necessary for any modification or constructive direction. To process interaction involves being able to reflect upon and evaluate just-completed actions. A diagram of this reflective characteristic of processing appears in Figure 12-2. As the diagram indicates, to process interaction means to pause and make a reflective "loopback" regarding what has just occurred (#1). The processing function of leadership means that people must be able to engage in this continuous reflective appraisal.

For example, suppose we are dealing with a group of nurses who are learning a new technique as part of their in-service training program. As we participate with the group in learning this technique, we also attend to the ongoing interaction that exists within the group. We may observe, for example, that some of the nurses recently out of school are already familiar with the technique, while several who received their training many years earlier are not familiar with it. We may also note that these older nurses, who occupy a higher-status position within the hospital staff, resent being put into a learning situation in which they are at a disadvantage relative to their more knowledgeable, younger colleagues. This resentment is expressed in many subtle ways: e.g., low attention on their part to the instruction; frequent and somewhat inappropriate joking; negativistic comments toward the whole procedure; tendency to avoid interacting with the younger nursing staff; resistance to being paired with younger staff in learning exercises. Processing, in this case, involves reflecting back on the interaction that is emerging while the teaching session itself occurs.

The interpersonal skills that also comprise the processing function require the leader to intervene appropriately in giving the group feedback based on this reflective evaluation. That is, the leader must continuously monitor the group in here-and-now terms. The information obtained from monitoring (#2) must be fed back to the group so that it can become a useful resource in the group's ongoing deliberations and interaction (#3). Inter-personal skills are demanded at this point. Having noted some critical aspect of the group's functioning, in what ways can the leader feed this information back to the group so that it becomes a resource for the group, something it can use to facilitate or transform its continuing behavior?

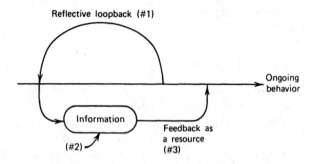

Figure 12-2. Processing the here and now.

The issue facing the group leader in our example is how to provide the group her perceptions regarding their mode of interacting together as a group. Should she simply interrupt the class and inform everyone about what she has seen? Or should she keep quiet and assume that learning will some-how occur regardless of how the group members seem to be relating to one another and to the new technique to be mastered? Should the leader con-front one of the senior nurses who seems to be the most resistant, saying something like, "You seem to be openly negativistic about this whole proce-dure; do you have any sense of why this might be?"

To the extent that the ongoing behavior of the group thwarts accom-plishment of its goals (in the example, by frustrating the learning of the new technique), the processing function of leadership requires: (a) perception of this ongoing pattern of group interaction, (b) evaluation of its role in help-ing or hindering the group, and (c) feedback of this appraisal so that it may be a resource the group can use to correct itself and thereby better accom-plish the goals. We will shortly examine both these cognitive and interper-sonal aspects of the processing function of leadership in greater detail.

SINGLE-LOOP VS. DOUBLE-LOOP LEARNING

Argyris (1975; 1976; Argyris & Schon, 1974) contrasts what he terms single-loop with double-loop behavior; the skills of double-loop learning are those that involve what we have termed the processing functions of leadership.

The example that Argyris chooses to illustrate single-loop behavior is the thermostat, which adjusts the temperature in a room to match a pre-set figure: e.g., 72 degrees. The thermostat receives information from the room, checks that information against the pre-set figure, and feeds the information back so as to turn the heat on or off. In this manner it serves the function of keeping the room at its temperature goal, correcting deviations as necessary. It may appear that this single-loop function is the critical key to good leadership. But Argyris suggests that double-loop behavior is even more important. In this latter case, the thermostat not only evaluates the degree to which the room temperature is on or off its designated target, but goes one step further; it evaluates the target itself. That is, a double-loop thermostat (if one were to exist) would also continuously evaluate whether a room temperature of 68°, 72°, or whatever was a reasonable goal.

Let us not get stuck in describing thermostats. Double-loop behavior within a group requires that the entire context within which the group functions be taken into consideration: that is, evaluation must be continuously made and fed back regarding the variety of alternative goals toward which the group might be heading, the variety of means whereby such goals can be achieved, the variety of consequences that follow from each alternative, the relation between each goal and the members' values, ethics, and responsibilities, and so forth.

Single-loop leader behavior within a group is concerned primarily with how well the group is moving toward a designated goal. This is relevant in many contexts, for example, when there is but one goal and no alternatives to be considered. However, in the usual circumstance, single-loop behavior will only inform the group regarding its deviation from one set goal. A double-loop perspective is needed for the introduction of multiple goals, alternatives, evaluations, and so forth.

Processing thereby involves being able to see where a group is heading, what alternatives are available, what their consequences are, how they may best be achieved, what members feel about these possibilities. All of this must be done while the group is engaged in its activities together; it must all be fed back to the group in order to become a further resource for members' consideration. This is a critical point.

To summarize, we are saying that an important leadership function and skill involves being able to help the group process itself *as it is behaving*. This involves providing a continuous flow of feedback to the group regarding its present situation and the multiplicity of futures toward which it can head. This continuous flow of feedback becomes an additional resource for the group. Knowledge about where it is, where it is going, and where it might be going becomes further material that a group can use in moving most effectively to achieve those ends that it deems essential. And one of the most important functions of leadership involves facilitating this ongoing processing of group behavior.

THE PERCEPTUAL AND INTERPERSONAL
SKILLS OF PROCESSING

LEADER: Let's stop for a few minutes now and take a look at our meeting today. We will want to see if we can describe what has gone on here, to analyze what we have done and how we feel about it. We may also want to take some time to make suggestions for changes that we would like to see.

MEMBER J: I noted that you (pointing to the leader) tried on several occasions to get us to summarize the points we had been making; but for the most part we seemed to ignore that and just continue with the particular point we wanted to make.

MEMBER L: I think that we aren't yet ready to summarize; we first need to develop more points and explore them.

MEMBER K: Yes. There are a lot of details and a lot of points still to be made; but I think we should pause now and try to summarize where we have been. I know that it helps me to know what ground I've covered before trying to move ahead.

MEMBER N: You know, I was so involved in what we were talking about that I just didn't think to stop and check on where we were and where we wanted to go.

LEADER: You see, I wasn't certain how to help in this. I felt a bit confused, with so many ideas and suggestions being made. I felt that we needed to stop and try to take stock before going on. Do you have any suggestions you can make to ensure that we build in this feedback and evaluation rather than just going on and not reflecting on our process?

This leader is attempting to help the group process its previous interaction before it continues. In this case, the leader's feedback to the group is the suggestion that members stop and review before moving ahead. The skills required of this leader include both perceptual and interpersonal abilities.

Perceptual Skills and Processing

Before leaders can intervene in the group and help members evaluate their present situations and their future possibilities, they must be able to *perceive* the unfolding ongoing situation. This requires that leaders be able to view themselves and the group with some perspective. As a full participant within the middle of interaction it becomes difficult to see just what is going on. The leader must adopt a somewhat more distant and analytic role, typically referred to as that of *participant-observer*. The leader both participates in the group and at the same time observes his or her own and others' participation. We can represent this in the following diagram (Fig. 12-3).

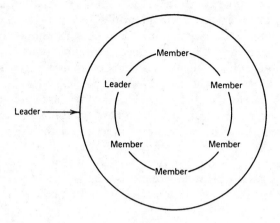

Figure 12-3. Perceiving as a participant-observer.

Dual Roles and Interests

The diagram illustrates the dual roles and perceptual interests of group leaders who serve the processing function: they are simultaneously within the group as a member and outside the group as an observer viewing themselves and the entire group. One must be inside the group in order to fully understand and appreciate what is being said and experienced by group members; yet one must also be outside the group looking in to see the interaction with some detachment and perspective.

The observer is attentive to patterns of interaction that can be visible only with distance and perspective, e.g. noting that whenever Mary speaks to George, she acts in a deferential manner; or that Sally seems to insist on calling attention to herself, thereby drawing the group away from its other activities in order to attend to Sally. Observers are attentive to the here and now situation. They must actively attempt to see, to experience, and to think in terms of what is taking place here and now. And they must remember that they are part of that here-and-now process.

For example, the leader observes that one member of the group is being negativistic; his actions keep the group fighting and disagreeing. Other members appear restless; one or two express a minor degree of irritation. While noting this behavior, the leader also begins to feel anger arising within herself; the anger is directed toward the negativistic member. Thus, the leader notes something about herself and something about her group: she occupies two roles with two perceptual interests at the same time. It is precisely at this point that the leader requires knowledge of the group process. She must be sensitive to group structures and processes, to theories of group formation and development, to verbal and nonverbal modes of communication.

The good observer is a theoretically informed observer.

People generally have difficulty with the idea that they are both participant and observer, occupying dual roles with dual perceptual interests at the same time. The temptation for many persons who work with groups is to adopt one role with only one perceptual interest. Thus, for example, some elect to be all participant and abandon their observer status; others elect to be all observer and abandon their participant status. The former lose a chance to facilitate the group process; they become so caught up in the interaction that they are unable to have the distance necessary to see what is taking place. The latter lose a chance to use their own feelings and experiences as a basis for a better, often more profound understanding of what is taking place in the group. In the example, the leader's awareness of her own anger was a helpful piece of information about the impact of the negativistic member's behavior on herself and on others in the group.

Interpersonal Skills and Processing: Feedback

The leader may be a keen observer; he may be informed and knowledgeable about group process. Yet if his observations and knowledge are to be anything more than of private or abstract theoretical concern, he must be able to translate this information into a resource that the group as a whole can use. The leader in the dialogue at the beginning of this section not only has made observations and analyses of the group, but has also sought to intervene by feeding this material back into the group. They were asked to stop and to review before continuing; in addition, they were asked to develop some procedure for making a review a regular part of their group. In other words, the leader sought to help the group answer several kinds of questions:

1. Where have we been in our discussion thus far?
2. Where do we want to take our discussion?
3. How can we work to ensure that we will ask and answer these questions throughout our future discussions?

In providing this feedback to the group, this leader did not seek to direct the group as such; she sought to provide members with information regarding their whereabouts based on her explicit observations and concerns. This leader, using the democratic style, feels that providing feedback to the group will be sufficient to help members improve themselves and their group. That is, she sees her role as being primarily to introduce questions that cause members to focus on their own process of interaction; the assumption is that they can then take this material and use it effectively.

Hypothesis Testing

Another quality of this leader's feedback should be noted. She offers her suggestions in the form of questions and hypotheses that she is testing for their validity. She does not make the assumption that she has the correct appraisal but only that this is her assessment of the group's status. She asks to have her view validated against the views of the others. Her feedback is of the double-loop variety; it is bilateral rather than unilateral as with single-loop behavior. This leader does not *steer* the group, but provides it with ideas to be tested, challenged, and critically evaluated. For example, it is her impression that they should stop and evaluate where they have been; others may disagree. It is her suggestion that they try to build in some procedure for ongoing evaluation; others may disagree.

It may appear that pausing to process a group's behavior takes valuable time away from the important business at hand. Time, to be sure, is not a luxury that we can spend freely. Some groups do not have the time to pause and reflect before acting. In the long run, however, quality solutions to difficult problems and acceptance of decisions hinge on the ability of a group to delay its headlong rush toward a goal before it has processed its movement toward that goal. It may appear impractical to pause. But there is hardly anything as impractical as rushing to a judgment that no one can accept, no one can really agree with, no one really wants to implement, and most importantly from which no one learns enough to become more proficient in group work the next time around.

INTERPERSONAL SKILLS AND PROCESSING: SOME BASIC TECHNIQUES

The main characteristic of processing is to provide feedback to individuals or to the group about behavior and its effects. It is assumed that this feedback can become a resource which the individual or group can use to help evaluate its ongoing actions and make whatever adjustments are felt to be necessary in order to function more effectively. This is an important assumption. We assume that if people could be more aware of their actions and the consequences of these actions, they could use this information to work more effectively. This assumption is reasonable in most cases; there is no guarantee, however, that sheer awareness will always be effective in producing needed change. Yet without awareness and knowledge of behavior and its effects, there is little chance to adjust and improve individual or group performance.

An Example of the Feedback Process

Feedback, the crux of processing, can be directed toward an individual member as well as to the group as a whole. For example, the leader may notice that whenever Harry speaks in the group, he lowers his voice, averts his gaze downward, shifts his chair, and leans away from others. The leader may also notice that Harry's ideas, though often sound and helpful for the group to consider, are rarely listened to and never openly discussed. It is as though

Harry were not present even though he participates frequently. The leader may feed these perceptions back both to Harry and to the group: "I've noticed, Harry, that whenever you speak you look downward, your voice gets very soft and difficult to hear, and you lean away from the rest of us. This gives me the impression that you lack confidence in your suggestions or are fearful about having others respond to them. I notice myself therefore tending to ignore or at least not pay much attention to what, on reflection, I think are some good ideas. I've also noticed that others in the group respond to you in this same way. That is, your ideas are not examined or discussed. It is difficult for a group to work with someone's ideas when the person proposing them seems to be so fearful that to challenge or to examine them closely would be a frightening thing. I wonder if others feel this way and if there is something that we can do about this?"

In this example, the leader provides feedback to Harry and to the group. The feedback follows a useful model for both leaders and other members to learn; the model involves asking and providing answers to four key questions:

1. What do I see?
    The feedback concretely describes a behavior or pattern of behavior that has been observed: e.g., looking downward, soft voice, leaning away.

2. How does it affect me?
    The feedback describes the effect of this behavior on the leader and its possible effect on the group as a whole: e.g., we tend to ignore what are probably some good ideas.

3. Is this perception and its effects shared by others?
    The feedback presents the leader's observations as hypotheses that need to be checked against the perceptions of others: e.g., do others feel this way?

4. What can we do about it?
    The feedback opens the door to using the information as a resource for continued work and problem-solving: e.g., given these observations, what can we all do to change the undesirable situation?

In the example, the leader's impressions were shared by several other group members; they indicated that often they had wanted to respond to Harry but felt his shyness put them off; they were fearful that if they questioned him closely about his suggestions he would be unable to handle things. Harry, in turn, became aware of his behavior and was able to reassure the group that he was strong enough to take criticism—in fact, that he was eager to have the group work with some of his ideas. Both he and the group were able to alter their behavior sufficiently to begin to use Harry's ideas in the group. To be sure, his manner did not suddenly change; he did not become a bold speaker. Rather, he became aware of the manner by which he presented his ideas; he was able to monitor his own behavior and thus could make adjustments accordingly. The group members, in turn, made special efforts to listen to Harry and to critically discuss his ideas. He did not crack under this new challenge, but rather grew more confident about himself and his contributions.

Processing involves giving feedback to individuals or to the group using the four key elements we noted. But what are the various techniques that are available for giving this feedback? We outline and briefly examine several major techniques. In each case, the goal of the technique remains much the same: to provide information about ongoing behavior and its effects so that this information can become a resource for persons to evaluate and use to modify their actions to better accomplish their goals and interests.

Support

Support involves giving the kind of feedback that helps a person or group continue with its ongoing actions by providing a climate of supportive opinion for this continuation. A supportive intervention for the entire group, for example, may be something as simple as the leader's statement: "I think that we are really doing well now; we seem to be working very effectively, generating some excellent proposals and critically examining each."

Unfortunately, we often mistakenly believe that the only proper kind of feedback involves being critical and informing people when they are off target; with support, however, we recognize that much learning can come from being informed about those times when we are on target. The leader can support an individual member by using positive comments to reinforce useful or helpful behavior, e.g., "Mary's suggestion that we reconsider our early proposal seems to me to be a good idea. I'm not sure that we'll act any differently on it now than we originally did, but it makes good sense for us to stop and reevaluate some of our earlier ideas in light of where we now are. That was a good idea, Mary."

Supportive comments serve several functions:

1. They inform persons about behaviors that at least the leader feels are on target and helpful; in this way they permit members to learn when they are doing well.

2. They create a climate of greater confidence for expressing unpopular ideas. None of us really wishes to stand forth with suggestions that others will ridicule or reject offhand. A supportive comment can facilitate the expression of unpopular ideas that may indeed gain in popularity once they are expressed. This is a critical function of leadership: to provide a climate within which divergent points of view can be expressed. Much of this climate is produced in and through the use of supportive comments e.g., "I know that your idea is not popular with this group, but I, for one, am really pleased that

you made it. I think it is a kind of thing that we need more of. I'm not sure yet how I feel about your suggestion, but I do know I'm glad you made it and that we can now all consider it."

3. They help the silent or the more fearful members feel that if they speak in the group there will be someone who will recognize and respond to them. Thus, by being supportive, the leader can facilitate greater member participation.

Confrontation

This is a nasty word, one that brings quickly to mind aggressive battles and warfare. Nothing is farther from the truth about confrontation, however. When we confront someone in the group, we do not intend to do battle or wage war; our goal is not aggressive; we do not wish to conquer. Our goal is, as with all forms of proper feedback, to be helpful in presenting behavior and its effects to the individual or the group. Confrontation is a challenge, however; it tends to startle individuals by forcing them to realize something about themselves and their behavior that they might not otherwise have noted or wanted to note. When we confront people, we place them in a sense in front of a mirror—our perceptions of them—and insist that they look into that mirror and see what they might not otherwise wish to see. We can confront an individual or the group as a whole.

For example, the leader may have noted that one member, Jane, seems insistent in taking the group away from its task and onto off-target discussions. Whenever the discussion seems to get going, Jane is sure to be on hand with something else that she would like everyone to talk about. And, given the difficulties in getting started and remaining on target, everyone else seems to delight in conspiring with Jane to discuss matters that avoid their important but difficult tasks at hand. The leader directly confronts Jane with her behavior: "Jane. I think it is important for you and for the rest of us to stop for a moment and consider what you are doing. It is my impression that whenever we get going in our discussion, for some reason you take us on a side trip. You seem unable or unwilling to let us remain on target or to help us remain on target. I think this is something we should stop and deal with." Here the leader directly confronts Jane with her behavior and invites her and the group to consider it further.

Groups and individuals often get themselves trapped into a pattern of interaction that is undesirable but that they refuse or are unable to see and thus cannot deal with. They cannot get themselves out of this trap because they fail even to see that they are in one in the first place. In the previous example, the group's task involved the discussion of a particularly difficult case, one that challenged the competency of the medical and nursing staff and thus, one they preferred not to have to deal with. They found Jane's off-target commentary helpful in letting them avoid what they feared. To help them realize their denial and avoidance, the leader confronted them directly:

e.g., "I think that this group is not sure about how to deal with this case. It's the kind of challenge that makes us aware of our own uncertainties as health professionals and so we prefer to avoid discussing it. We joke; we laugh nervously; we let Jane lead us into digressions. I feel that in pointing this out, I'm violating an implicit understanding that we not openly deal with this troublesome case. But I believe that this is a hurdle that we must overcome."

Confrontation and Support

The combination of *confrontation and support* can be one of the most effective change-inducing feedback techniques. Without confrontation—that is, without introducing some doubt, tension, or challenge into the system— there is little likelihood of change. And yet, without a supportive climate to reassure and build confidence, confrontation is likely to result in defensiveness rather than in learning. The leader who would only confront is thereby not likely to be helpful in permitting groups or individuals to learn from their behavior; defensiveness results. Likewise, the leader who is only supportive, who never introduces challenges that produce growth and that drive us to reevaluate our existing ways of behaving, is not likely to help the group or its members move forward as far as they might. The combination of confrontation and support is an important set of techniques for the leader which serves processing functions.

Advice and Suggestions

It almost goes without saying that one type of leadership intervention involves offering advice or suggestions to individuals or the group. The leader may have greater expertise and knowledge than members or may have a perspective on events that members do not have. Feedback that involves advice or suggestions can be helpful. It must be remembered, however, that we are talking about suggestions and advice and not directives. The goal is not to have members simply follow the leader's suggestions without subjecting them to critical evaluation; rather, it is to provide information that members or individuals can use once they have critically examined and evaluated it.

Summarizing

A team at a large urban hospital was observed at several of its meetings. The observer noted that the material at each meeting was brought up over and over again without any apparent resolution. She also noted that there were no summaries provided at the conclusion of any meeting, nor did the leader prepare a summary statement of the staff's still unresolved issues to open the next meeting. At her request, the team voted to take turns in summarizing each meeting before they ended and in preparing and presenting a listing of unresolved issues at the opening of their next meeting. As a result, the team members felt less frustrated; they were now able to make decisions which they could readily implement.

One of the most useful techniques of processing either individual or group behavior involves putting things together in a summary fashion. In doing this, the leader takes a range of behaviors over some period of time, and organizes and summarizes them for the group. Or, as in the example, the leader may ask the group to engage in its own summarization of what has taken place during a certain period. In either case, the goal of this intervention technique is to place an organized, summary statement of its immediately past action before the group.

For example, the leader can suggest that it will be helpful for the group to spend the last five minutes of its meeting reviewing and summarizing the meeting. The leader may then undertake this review and summary or may have members reconstruct the meeting. This reconstruction can focus on decisions that were made, problems that were confronted, issues still before the group that must be considered for the next meeting, and so forth. In the rush of a day's work and in our interests to get our job done, we often forget how useful it can be simply to pause and review where we have just been, what we have just done, and where we plan to head in our next discussion.

Furthermore, in order to summarize, we must organize our recollections of events just past. In the very process of organizing. we may become aware of things that we had not otherwise considered; we may see relationships among events that we would otherwise have ignored. In other words, the very process of attempting to provide a summary for a meeting can offer new insights and new perspectives on things that have already taken place.

Clarification

So much human communication gets distorted and confused in its movement between the transmitter and receiver that an extremely useful leadership function can be served by having either the leader or members directly clarify what has been said. The goal of this intervention is to check on the meanings of the interaction and communication. Leaders, for example, may ask members to clarify their remarks: e.g., "I'm not certain just what you meant when you stated that you find John's analysis of the case in error. Could you tell us what you mean?" Or, they may attempt their own clarification: e.g., "What I heard you saying is that you disagree with John's analysis of the case. Is that correct?"

Through clarification, the leader hopes to help the group better understand itself and its communications. In recognition of the often needlessly confusing consequences of misunderstandings, the leader's aim is to help clarify communications that could be misunderstood before members can react to the misunderstandings. There is enough difficulty resulting from real conflicts of interest and clashes of different value systems. This is substantive conflict that a group should confront and work on. Needless conflict, however, is based on faulty communication in transmission or reception. Through clarifying interventions, the leader hopes to minimize the detrimental impact of these kinds of needless and nonsubstantive conflicts.

For example, John and Bill basically agree in what they are saying but fail to hear and to understand each other. By clarifying what has been said, the leader hopes to make it possible for them to see that they are really agreeing. By asking members to clarify what they mean (e.g., "I'm not sure I understand what you just said or meant") and by taking the role of clarifier (e.g., "This is what I hear you saying..."), the leader intervenes to facilitate more accurate communication within the group.

Probing and Questioning

Probing and questioning are techniques that trained interviewers learn. Through these methods the respondent is pressed for more information, more material, so that a better understanding or a deeper insight is made possible. Probing and questioning are useful process interventions in group leadership. The leader may probe by directly asking a question: e.g., "You just said that Dr. Williams' approach is something that you find helpful. Could you tell us more about what in his technique you find valuable?" The probe might take a less direct form: e.g., "A new technique?" In this latter example, often the repetition of the last few comments made by a member will serve to trigger a continuation of the member's commentary.

Through probing and questioning the leader hopes to help members generate more material concerning their ideas and opinions. It is not unusual for members simply to state an opinion or viewpoint and leave it at that. This provides little for others to work with; and so the leader may use probing and questioning to get more material out before the group to consider and to evaluate. For example, a member might say in response to another's comments: "No, I don't think that's a good idea". That statement may be made with such finality that there is little that the group can do other than to go on to another member or another issue. But the perceptive leader might probe and question in order to turn that final period into a comma: e.g., "I wish you could tell us more about your own thoughts on this matter; it would be helpful for us to hear more from you."

A Caution

Probing by an inexperienced leader can backfire and produce high anxiety in a group or in a member. Improperly done, probing and questioning can make people feel they are being "grilled" or challenged. The idea behind a probe is to help persons say more fully what they know and wish to share; a probe should usually not be used to force people to disclose things that they wish to keep secret; nor should questions be used improperly to make people feel stupid or incompetent. These are some of the pitfalls of probing that the inexperienced leader may inadvertently implement.

A Guide to Better Probing

Given some of the problems that improper probing can produce, it is helpful for the leader to use this type of intervention with caution. When questioning and probing are employed there are certain helpful guides for handling the situation. For example, one way of getting more from the speaker is simply to say, "Could you expand a bit further on what you've just said?" This invites more information and gives the person freedom to say no or to go on. When we next consider the technique called repetition, we will note another way to probe for more material without grilling the person. For example, the leader can simply repeat the last few words of the speaker:

SPEAKER: I'm not sure that we should pursue this matter any further.
LEADER: You're not sure about pursuing it?
SPEAKER: Well, there is just one more thing I'd like to talk about here.

Basically, the intent of the probing and questioning technique is to help group members develop and expand on something they are saying. The ideal is to help them do this when they are *ready* to, and about a matter or topic they are *willing* to examine further. Probing is not intended to push people to do something they don't want or aren't ready to do. Probing and question-ing, in the hands of the experienced group leader, are more like *invitations* to continue.

Repeating, Paraphrasing, Highlighting

Strictly speaking, repeating, paraphrasing, and highlighting are not differ-ent techniques as much as they are components of several of the preceding interventions. They offer the leader a more complete repertoire of process interventions that help provide feedback. The simple act of repeating often facilitates communication among group members. The leader simply repeats back what he or she has heard; this can serve to correct inaccurate commu-nication or emphasize accurate communication.

In the example we used to examine probing, we saw how the repetition of the speaker's words (e.g., "You're not sure about pursuing it?") were help-ful in allowing the speaker to decide on the direction of the conversation and to continue or to stop. One of the problems that less experienced leaders often run into is the tendency to lose the speaker's thoughts and intent by placing their own meaning onto it. Thus the leader, not the speaker, decides on the direction of the conversation and we learn more about the leader's concerns than the member's. For example:

MEMBER: I'm not sure that we should pursue this project.
LEADER: Are you afraid that we'd run into the same difficulty here as on our last case?
MEMBER: No, I hadn't thought of that; but now that you mention it, perhaps . . .

What has happened here is that the leader has implanted a doubt or anxiety (one that may well be her own) and has lost the member's own thoughts. Repetition can help avoid or at least minimize that possibility:

> MEMBER: I'm not sure that we should pursue this project.
> LEADER: You're not sure that we should pursue this project?
> MEMBER: That's right. I think it is very foolish of us to think that with our small numbers and lack of facilities we can bring about such a large change as we've proposed.

Note how the repetition has brought the member's own thoughts to light without the improper interposition of the leader's particular worries.

In paraphrasing, the leader hopes to clarify matters by repeating what has been said, but as a paraphrase rather than as a direct repetition. For example, a member might say, "I'm not sure just how we should go about dealing with Mrs. French's family; sometimes I think we'd be better off if we could deal with her and leave her family out of the picture entirely." A paraphrase might take this form: "You're puzzled about what we should do with Mrs. French's family." The purpose of this paraphrase is to *highlight* what the leader senses to be the main thrust of the member's comments. In this way, the group can focus on the main issue and not get overly involved in side issues. At the same time, when the leader's perception of the important element in the member's communication is highlighted, the member can respond with agreement or disagreement. In either case, there has been clarification; communication can flow more accurately within the group.

We should note that in paraphrasing or in highlighting, the leader is offering his or her version of what has been said. This is less likely with repetition. The more the paraphrase or the highlight is removed from what has been said, the more it becomes like an interpretation. We mention this not to discourage leaders from paraphrasing or highlighting, but to caution them that in some cases they are beginning to walk on the territory of interpretation and analysis.

Reflection

In reflecting, the leader focuses the attention of the individual or the group on the important feelings that are being communicated or on the behaviors that are taking place. Thus there are two related, though distinct, types of reflection: of feelings and of behaviors. We will examine each of these.

Reflection of Feelings

An example will help our understanding of the use of reflection of feelings:

> MEMBER: I've been working here for many, many years and I think that I know pretty much about proper procedures and things like that. I'm getting

tired of hearing from those new, young, fresh-from-college types about the right and proper way we should be doing things around here.

The leader might reflect back to this member and to the others in the group what feelings he or she thinks are being conveyed:

LEADER: You sound upset and annoyed with these young people.

In this type of intervention, the leader orients the members to the feelings that lie behind the content of the person's remarks. In this way, that person is allowed to deal with these feelings directly instead of passing them by as though they did not exist. For example, without the leader's intervention, the response to those comments might have been: "Well, we must get on with our main task today." Other members might avoid dealing with the feelings that lie behind the remarks. The leader, sensing that these feelings are important for the group to consider before continuing, uses reflection as a technique to bring the feelings to the focus of the group.

It need not only be an individual's feelings that are reflected, however; the leader may reflect feelings that are more generally shared, though unstated, among the group.

A nurse is working with a parent group in the community that is concerned with issues of sexuality. She is introducing her lecture on the anatomy and physiology of male and female sexual functioning and notices that there is much giggling and uneasiness among group members.

The nurse can either continue with her lecture, completely ignoring the parents' uneasiness, or she can intervene at this point by reflecting their feelings to them: e.g., "I sense that many of you are made anxious by this discussion. Perhaps this is something we should talk about before I continue with the lecture itself."

In the reflection of feelings, the leader searches behind the content of communications and responds to the feelings that are being conveyed either by *what* is said or by *how* it is said. Members may be talking about matters that on the surface seem to be nonemotional in content. The leader, however, notices some nonverbal behavior that suggests that there are strong feelings behind the mask of apparently neutral content. Lou says to Sam, in an apparently calm manner, "What you say is interesting, but I'm not sure that I can agree fully with you about it." The leader may notice that there is anger being communicated nonverbally: e.g., Lou's face tightens, her hands form a fist, she leans forward in an aggressive stance. These tell the leader about Lou's feelings. The leader then reflects these feelings: e.g., "I sense that you are very angry with Sam." These feelings can now become a focus for consideration.

Reflection of Behavior

In reflecting individual or group behavior, the leader engages in less interpretation than is usually involved when reflecting feelings. Thus, for example, the nurse working with the parent group might simply have reflected to them the fact that they are giggling and stirring about restlessly in their chairs. She may have then asked them what this could mean. The reflection of behavior involves informing the members what behavior the leader sees them carrying out: this will include nonverbal behavior of which the member may be aware or unaware (e.g., "I notice much restless moving about in the chairs"). It will also include verbal behaviors as in the following example:

MEMBER: I'm not sure what is expected of me around here; you old-timers seem to know what is going on; I'm still wet behind the ears; you old hands surely have better skills than I do; I'm fresh from college.

LEADER: I've noticed the words you use to describe yourself and the words you use to describe the others. They are all "old timers" and "old hands" and you're "still wet behind the ears." Could you tell us what you are feeling about being in this group?

As this example indicates, the leader has reflected back the member's actual *behavior* to him—in this case, the words he used in describing or explaining something. The leader, however, could also have reflected back the member's *feelings* to him: e.g., "You sound upset and anxious with your status as a new person in a group of experienced people."

Notice however, that to reflect feelings requires greater degree of interpretation than to reflect behaviors. The leader must be sensitive to this important distinction. Telling members what you see them doing or hear them saying is different than telling them what feelings you *think* they are expressing by what they are doing and saying. The former is more directly observational; the latter more interpretative and inferential. We are suggesting that the reflection of feelings should be done with great care and with a genuine openness to being incorrect.

Interpretation and Analysis

Interpretative interventions go several steps beyond sheer observation of individual or group behavior. The observations that the leader makes are placed within a theoretical context that gives them meaning; it is this meaning that is then fed back to the group or individual. The following is a brief illustration of interpretation as distinct from several of the other techniques we have considered:

GROUP MEMBER: I feel terrible about missing so many group meetings. (He speaks softly and hesitantly; his head is lowered; his brow is knitted; he bites his lips and wrings his hands.)

LEADER PARAPHRASING: Yes, you have missed several meetings.

LEADER REPEATING: You feel terrible about having missed so many meetings?

LEADER PROBING: Frankly, I was puzzled about your behavior. Why did you miss so many meetings?

LEADER REFLECTING FEELING: You sound rather upset and worried.

LEADER REFLECTING BEHAVIOR: While telling us this, your face is lowered, your brow is tightly knit, you are rubbing your hands together, and your voice is soft and hesitant. How you feeling?

LEADER CONFRONTING: It seems to me that having missed so many meetings must make it difficult for you to participate actively in this group. Just what do you plan to do about it?

LEADER INTERPRETING: I am beginning to wonder about why you have missed so many of our meetings or if there is a pattern to your absences. Although I'm not sure, I wonder if you are asking us to pay more attention to you but are asking this in a way that actually works to your disadvantage? (Schulman, 1974, offers a similar example.)

The leader's interpretation takes the observation of several absences and looks for some underlying pattern that gives meaning to that behavior. The meaning comes from locating the behavior in a larger theoretical context; that is, a particular behavior is rendered meaningful by virtue of its fitting into a theory. This is one reason why leaders must have clear understanding of theory in order to be able to intervene with interpretive or analytic comments.

In the example, the interpretation suggests that the member, for some reason, has need for more attention from the group and has used a nonproductive manner of seeking that attention, as if to say: "You'll really notice me when I'm not here." As the leader notes, excessive absence produces just the opposite effect; the member becomes even more distanced from the group and receives less and less attention.

The interpretive intervention is designed to help the member see his behavior from a new perspective. The hope is that this new view will help him gain better conscious control over his behavior and effect a change in it. That is, if the member really wants more attention, he must see that absences are not an effective way to get it. We leave out of this consideration the reasons why so much attention is needed; rather, we focus on the behavior and one level of interpretation; in this case, the aim is to help the person see that his goals are not being achieved by that particular behavior.

Let us take another example. Fran is a member who frequently says that she wants to be accepted and liked by others in her group. And yet, when she interacts with others, she continually interrupts them, cuts them off in mid-sentence, only rarely supports and agrees with them, and in any number of other ways seems to reject the very persons she says she wants to have accept her. The leader may choose to make an interpretive intervention:

> Fran—I've heard you say on several occasions that you are concerned about being liked and accepted by this group. And yet, I watch your behavior and notice that you tend to be abrupt, to interrupt others, to be overly critical of their comments, rarely to support or agree with them. You seem to me to act in ways that will not get others to like you or accept you. This leads me to wonder why you're doing this. I wonder if perhaps you so fear being rejected that you reject others before they have a chance either to accept or to reject you?

There are several features of this interpretation that need to be noted.

1. It summarizes Fran's past behavior and presents this summary to her. Thus it is an interpretation that is rooted to concrete behaviors. This helps Fran better see what there is about her and her behavior that call be corrected if she chooses or is able to do so.

2. It offers an analysis of Fran's behavior and what may be a deeper reason or meaning for it. In this case, the analysis is provided by a theoretical perspective that suggests that acceptance/rejection is an important issue for all of us; that, in fear of being rejected by others, some of us act to reject these others first. In this way we avoid discovering whether or not we are worthy of acceptance by creating our own conclusion.

3. This level of interpretation, though several steps removed from our observations, is not as deep an analysis as we could make. That is, the leader does not seek to probe much further beneath the surface to understand the whys and wherefores of Fran's fear of rejection or why she rejects before she is rejected.

The leader does not probe in order to understand some of the deeper bases for Fran's lack of self-esteem. The leader is content, rather, to focus on the actual behavior and some of its immediate consequences. We are not dealing with therapy or therapy groups in which interpretations that uncover more material at deeper levels of meaning may be necessary and important. In most groups, however, it is necessary to analyze in a way that will help members see the effects of their behavior; this lets them work to remedy those effects even though we and they may never attempt to get at the deeper causes that may persist. In the example, Fran can use the leader's interpretation to observe how her manner of interacting with others thwarts her gaining the acceptance she claims she so desperately wants. Thus, Fran can see that one of the consequences of her behavior is that it prevents her being accepted by others.

Group-Level Interpretations

Interpretations can also be made at the group level. For example, a consultant is called in to help a group diagnose and evaluate its difficulties. He observes that the group is led by a rather directive and autocratic leader; members fail to express any anger and resentment toward this leader. The consultant notices, however, that one member of the group seems to be the butt of jokes and criticisms, and is generally picked on excessively: i.e., this person's behavior does not seem to warrant his receiving the kind of treat-ment that he gets. From the consultant's perspective, this member appears to be the group's scapegoat, receiving all the angry and resentful feelings that members have toward their leader which they fear to express directly and openly.

The consultant decides to confront the group with this interpretation: "I've observed your meeting for some time now and have some impressions that I would like to share with you. First, I've noticed that Jerry seems to be the butt of much anger and resentment. As I watch his behavior, however, I have difficulty in seeing just what he's done to deserve all this anger. I wonder if perhaps there is some resentment that members have toward John, the group leader, that they are fearful of expressing and so have chosen Jerry as their scapegoat?"

There is no magic in this interpretive formulation. The members may respond with anger at the consultant, accusing him of coming in to mess up their otherwise happy group. The group leader may feel very threatened, not only by the consultant's presence in a challenging role but also by his interpretive remarks and their implication about his leadership style. Mem-bers may feel threatened by now having to consider directly and openly their hostilities toward their leader rather than continuing to use the faithful scapegoat, Jerry. They may now make the consultant their scapegoat. On the other hand, it is possible that the time is ripe for the group members to openly explore their behavior and that the consultant's interpretive intervention was just the catalyst they needed.

Listening

Good and attentive listening is perhaps one of the most important and critical processing approaches for leaders. Groups often become arenas for members simply to speak their piece without listening or responding to others. The process thus becomes somewhat like the parallel play of chil-dren, a loosely connected chaining of talkers none of whom pays attention to the others or to do more than minimally respond to others. The function of the leader as a listener can be critical.

In the first place, a listening leader gives members an attentive audience to whom they can address their remarks; it provides them someone who is responsive to what they say when no one else might be.

In the second place, the attentive, listening leader can help shape group process by *modeling* a desirable form of behavior. When leaders not only listen attentively with an aim to truly understanding what is being said and also act in ways that demonstrate this responsiveness—e.g., by responding appropriately to members' comments rather than by simply going off on their own track as others tend to do—then members can see the possibilities for their behaving in a similarly attentive and responsive manner.

Finally, an attentive and responsive listener can help speakers sharpen their own thinking and understanding. We all get sloppy in our speech and logic when we sense that no one is really listening or trying to understand us anyway. But the realization that there is someone who is both listening and trying to understand can force us to become more aware of just what we are saying. Although this may be somewhat inhibiting at first, in time listening can be highly instructive to members, especially when they make a concerted effort not only to talk in more communicative ways but also to become better listeners themselves.

Timing

If a cookbook of interpersonal skills could be written, surely it would specify precisely the proper timing for leader interventions. However, no serious student of group process would write a cookbook; it is just too complex a subject. Timing is the most critical and difficult lesson of all to learn. Regardless of the technique employed, the leader must choose intelligently and carefully the timing of any intervention. To intervene too soon by confronting or interpreting may elicit defensiveness. On the other hand, to let matters go and be allowed to build up pressure when they should have been dealt with earlier is not helpful either.

In other words, the leader might wish to "strike while the iron is hot" because "there is no better time than the present" or might properly sense that "silence is golden" and "discretion is the better part of valor." Proper timing involves a very sensitive assessment of the group and its situation. There are no hard and fast rules for definitive guidance. Experience can be an excellent teacher. In general, however, it is wise first to facilitate the creation of a supportive climate, one within which members feel secure enough with themselves and their leader to take some risks. The leader must explore the group's process *before* intervening with confrontation or interpretation.

Basically, the leader must remember that the goal is to help the group process its ongoing behavior so that members may work together more effectively. The leader must evaluate timing in terms of whether or not an intervention at a particular point will help the group better achieve its goals.

One of the best ways of learning about timing is to venture forth and try. Ask the group: "Are my comments timed to be as helpful as they might be?" Make a trial intervention. If there are loud denials or if people ignore you completely, then perhaps your timing is off. Wait and try again later.

Obviously, a group that is meeting only once must be dealt with differently than a group that meets on a continuing basis. The former cannot tolerate much process intervention; its members do not have the time to deal with complex interpretations, challenging confrontations, or reflections of feelings. A leader who intervenes to point out a process that must be worked on and evaluated by the group must realize that time is needed to do this work. It is poor and inappropriate timing therefore to intervene with process-type comments when there is no time or opportunity for members to follow up and evaluate what new doors and perspectives the leader has opened.

Time is needed to work on material that process interventions bring to light. Thus to intervene late in a session may be a poor idea—a summary might be more helpful at such a point. Likewise, just after a meeting has begun can be a bad time to interpret and to analyze, unless members have a past history of working effectively together in processing their ongoing actions.

RESISTANCE AND PROCESSING

Dr. Romero is the director of one of the hospital's units. He sets aside a half-hour each week for the staff members to "process" (his term) their own inter-personal material. At 2 P.M. sharp each Wednesday, after the staff has convened he says. "Well, what are our concerns this week?" The staff has great resistance to this processing of their own relationships. It is a new idea to most of them; it is frightening. For almost five months they have talked about how hard it is to do. A new member has joined the staff. She becomes quite angry during these sessions and keeps saying "You people don't dare examine your own rela-tionships as staff members or your feelings about Dr. Romero." The resistance does not decrease. But gradually. as tensions on the unit increase—primarily because administrative pressures are increasing and the severity of patients' illness is proving disturbing to most of the staff—they begin to test the idea of sharing. They begin to examine their relationship as staff members and note that their tensions, especially those from external sources (e.g., administration and patients) begin to diminish as they do this. The atmosphere on the entire unit begins to clear and lighten. Their resistance has faded considerably and they now almost eagerly await those weekly sessions.

As the example suggests, processing as a leadership function is by no means heartily accepted either by leaders or by group members. There are many bases for resistance to the processing function. It will help us to exa-mine four of these: (1) the difficulty in perceiving one's self behaving; (2) polite norms that shy away from examining ongoing behavior; (3) power plays and the tactics of winning that lead people to suspect the motives of those who would process and provide feedback; (4) the fear of looking foolish, acting inappropriately, or appearing weak.

Perceiving Ongoing Behavior

We should really not consider this first point as much a matter of resistance as a matter of a basic human difficulty. We cannot simultaneously behave and see ourselves behaving. To try to become conscious of ourselves behaving disrupts our performance. For example, we can read and we can write; but if we focus our attention on the actual process by which our reading or writing is taking place, it disrupts the reading or writing. However, we are able to stop and reflect back on what we have done; or we can use others as sources of information for our own activity.

Paradoxically, we are directly in touch with others at the moment of their behaving but are in touch with ourselves only *after* we have behaved (Schutz, 1970-1971). We see others directly and immediately and ourselves reflectively. We need those others, therefore, to keep us informed about our behavior and its effects. Their feedback plays a critical role in informing us about ourselves. Naturally, we can pause and reflect back on our own actions and thereby supply our own feedback. Or, as several efforts have demonstrated (e.g., Storms, 1973), we can use videotape to play back our own actions, giving us an observer's view of ourselves; but this is the kind of view we cannot obtain without a device such as a video recorder.

Whether we use others to give us feedback, pause and reflect on our own actions, or use some mechanical recording device, in all cases we need information about our actions in order to evaluate and adjust. We need feedback before we can function more effectively and learn how to improve the next time around. Groups are in a similar position. Members get so caught up in developing their own points of view that they cannot see what is going on or how their behavior contributes to the group's getting bogged down in detail when it needs to take stock of itself.

The difficulties we have in seeing ourselves behaving and interacting with others makes adjustment in our performances, and hence our learning, a real problem. We must openly court feedback from others, or pause frequently to reflect on ourselves, in order to modify our actions in light of the consequences they produce.

Social Norms

As several analysts have noted (e.g., Argyris, 1976; Yalom, 1975), it is not polite to process another person's behavior. Parents do it with their children, commenting on the ways they are behaving and the consequences of behaving in those ways: "You are shouting now; why are you so angry?" "Don't talk to me like that!" When adults call attention to these matters, we feel they are behaving impolitely. And yet, it is just this kind of normative violation that is required to fulfill the leadership function of processing. There cannot be any processing for a group unless people, both leaders and members, are willing to drop some of the polite norms that discourage their focusing on and reviewing ongoing behavior.

The typical response, however, when norms have been violated is to try to normalize the situation again. If one person processes what she believes is taking place, others may respond by angrily denying that anything is taking place other than what we have all seen or heard; or that the person doing the processing must be crazy; or they might try to ignore it all together and continue as though nothing had happened.

> NURSE ASH: Doctor Sells, I have the feeling that whenever you give me an order you do so with a kind of arrogance that says to me that either you are insecure about me or frightened of me, or something like that.
>
> DR. SELLS: I'm sure I don't know what you're talking about. Anyway, what does it matter? Your job is clear. Follow precisely what I say.
>
> NURSE ASH: It's not that. I'm not questioning your authority; I'm not even challenging your orders. I was just wondering if you felt some need to put me down by acting so arrogantly whenever you address me.
>
> DR. SELLS: That's stupid. Why would I want to do something like that! Now, let's get back to our rounds.

There are several important implications of the normative view of resistance. A leader must play an active part in helping create new norms. Or, the leader must support those members who are more willing than others to engage in processing, who are willing to violate norms that forbid its usage. Basically, the leader must help create an atmosphere in which processing and feedback are part of the normal and routine life of the group. A leader who would simply process without having created a normative climate for it or helping to explain its usefulness is simply asking for trouble, resistance, and rejection.

One way for the leader to help break down the resistant old norms and facilitate the emergence of norms that are most hospitable to processing is for the leader to ask for feedback about his or her own behavior. This can also help clear the way for others to engage in similar activities. It also makes the leader appear more human, vulnerable, and approachable.

Social Power

Unfortunately, processing and feedback are too often used as weapons of battle than as techniques for serious group self-evaluation. Many people process the behavior of others as a way to get back at them, to demean them, to put them down, to hurt them, to put them in their place, to score points, to win, or whatever. Understanding and self-correction are not the goal of this kind of processing; winning is.

For this reason people suspect processing; it makes the one processed more vulnerable and thereby triggers defenses. When we report people's behavior back to them, they tend not to be open and receptive to hearing about it; rather, they almost instinctively put up defenses, to deny it, to argue about it, or better still to pick on a piece of *our* behavior and cast it back quickly to put us off our guard. Processing in the name of winning and of garnering more power is not helpful to group interaction. However, processing that equalizes the vulnerability, that opens up the lines of communication, is useful. Thus leaders who court feedback on their own behavior make themselves more vulnerable; this now equalizes the vulnerability that members tend to experience and so can reduce resistance.

The motivations behind processing, therefore, must be clear in the minds of those who do it. If they are out to prove a point—their own, or make a point—their own, or score a point—their own, or demonstrate how perceptive and insightful they are, then they are not processing in the service of accomplishing effective group functioning. Their aims are not to help a group evaluate its course and its alternatives, but rather to demonstrate something about themselves and their relationships to others. They use processing as a weapon to gain or to maintain power over others.

Stated in another way, one who processes must be open to being processed. One cannot hope to feed information back into a group without thereby becoming a part of that group process. The contributor creates a position of vulnerability for himself or herself within the group. One cannot process as a spectator, as though casting the first stone and then rushing away; rather, one must process from inside and thereby become as vulnerable as everyone else. It is no wonder, then, that so many group leaders shy away from this kind of bilateral engagement, preferring to exercise their unilateral control and thereby avoid being vulnerable.

The beneficial function of processing requires the processor to be processed as well. The leader who asks the group to stop and evaluate itself must remember that he or she thereby is open to evaluation as well. It is not simply that the leader, from outside or on high, says, "You take a look at where you are and where you are going." From within the group, the leader says, "Let us take a look at ourselves, where we have been and where we are going. And let us look at the kind of leadership I am providing and how this too can be improved."

Fear

Because processing behavior places the leader and members on a more equal standing, opening up their relationship to examination and evaluation, many leaders, as we have noted, shy away from its use. They choose a more autocratic style and avoid any hints at processing, unless they see a way for it to be used unilaterally toward their own ends. But there is another leader-based resistance to processing: fear.

Argyris (1976) captures this fear perfectly in his discussion of a group of business executives who finally learned the perceptual and interpersonal skills of processing and became proficient in its use but who still were fearful of using it back home in their organizations. When probed about their reasons for this fear, it was discovered that they felt their subordinates would think them foolish, inappropriate, or weak as leaders. Quite a strong set of reasons not to put into practice the excellent leadership skills that they had just learned!

The terrible trio—foolish, inappropriate, and weak—consisted of precisely the feelings they had had when first entering the training course in which they learned how to engage in the processing functions of leadership. Their first sessions were spent in commenting on the foolishness of the business executive who asks others to reflect on their behavior with him; on the inappropriateness of this; of the weakness and vulnerability that it suggested. After all, only a weak leader would do anything other than dominate and lead with great confidence and self-assurance.

These fears are difficult to overcome; in fact, it is only through the use of processing that group leaders begin to experience its advantages and to experience themselves as stronger through its use and as weaker without.

Reflect for a moment on the possibility of leaders who dominate the discussion and direct others toward their ends vs. leaders who confidently open up their group and their leadership to frequent self-examination. Who are the more foolish, less appropriate, and weaker of the two? We suspect the self-confidence of leaders who would never examine their practice, who would never reflect with their group on its process, who would never wish to evaluate their own or their group's actions.

SUMMARY AND CONCLUSIONS

The functions of leadership require careful study and understanding of all the chapters that have preceded this one and a consideration of the material in the remaining chapter. Chapters artificially segment and isolate the kinds of knowledge and skills that must be woven together if one is to work effectively as a group leader or as a helpful and effective group member.

Table 12-1 provides a useful summary of the various types of leader interventions that we have covered in this chapter. The table indicates both the types that we have discussed and the important goals and functions each type is said to serve.

Table 12-1. A Summary of Leader Interventions

Type of Intervention	Goals of Intervention
Support	Provides supportive climate for expressing ideas and opinions, including unpopular or unusual points of view.
	Facilitates members continuing with their ongoing behavior.
	Helps reinforce positive forms of behavior.
	Creates a climate in which silent members may feel secure enough to participate.
Confrontation	Aids in growth and development; helps unfreeze members from being stuck in one mode of functioning.

Table 12-1. *(Continued)*

Type of Intervention	Goals of Intervention
	Helps reduce some forms of disruptive behavior.
	Helps members deal more openly and directly with each other.
Advice and Suggestions	Shares expertise, offers new perspectives.
	Helps focus group on its task and goals.
Summarizing	Helps keep group on its task by reviewing past actions and by setting agenda for future sessions.
	Brings to focus still unresolved issues.
	Organizes past in ways that help clarify; brings into focus themes and patterns of interaction.
Clarifying	Helps reduce distortion in communication.
	Facilitates focus on substantive issues rather than allowing members to be side-tracked into misunderstandings.
Probing and Questioning	Helps expand a point that may have been left incomplete.
	Gets at more extensive and wider range of information.
	Invites members to explore their ideas in greater detail.
Repeating, Paraphrasing, and Highlighting	Helps members continue with their ongoing behavior; invites further exploration and examination of what is being said.
	Clarifies and helps focus on the specific, important, or key aspect of a communication.
	Sharpens members' understanding of what is being said or done.
Reflecting: Feelings	Orients members to the feelings that may lie behind what is being said or done.
	Helps members deal with issues they might otherwise avoid or miss.
Reflecting: Behavior	Gives members the opportunity to see how

Table 12-1. A Summary of Leader Interventions

Type of Intervention	*Goals of Intervention*
	their behavior appears to others and to see and evaluate its consequences.
	Helps members to understand others' perceptions and responses to them.
Interpretation and Analysis	Renders behavior meaningful by locating it in a larger context in which a causal explanation is provided.
	Helps members understand both the likely bases of their behavior and its meaning.
	Summarizes a pattern of behavior and provides a useful way of examining it and working to modify it through the insights gained.
Listening	Provides an attentive and responsive audience for those who participate.
	Models a helpful way for members to relate to one another; gives a feeling of sharing and mutual concern.
	Helps members sharpen their own ideas and thinking as they realize that indeed others are listening and concerned about what they are saying.

13

Dealing with Specific Group Problems

The health professional who leads groups usually has many "how-to" questions about issues encountered in most groups. In this final chapter, we will examine seven issues that group leaders often confront:

1. Dealing with the member who dominates or monopolizes the discussion,

2. Dealing with the silent member or the apathetic-silent group,

3. Dealing with emotional outbursts such as anger or crying,

4. Dealing with group conflict,

5. Dealing with normative deviance, with behaviors that violate group norms and expectations for proper member behavior,

6. Dealing with the issues involved in beginning a group, and

7. Dealing with the issues involved in ending or terminating a group.

This chapter, by itself, without careful consideration of the material in the preceding chapters, can have an excessively mechanical quality to it. As with most skilled professional activities, technical competence, while important, does not make up the entire picture that is necessary for effective leadership. This chapter builds upon the work of the preceding chapters and assumes a general familiarity and understanding on the part of the reader of that work. Its "cookbook" appearance is deceptive. One cannot simply follow a recipe for group intervention techniques and get from here to there.

It is especially important for the practitioner to recognize that subtle interpersonal factors involving concern and empathy are as important for the group leader as the skills with which this chapter primarily deals. Likewise, a solid grounding in group process theory is a prerequisite to effective leadership. Technical skills for intervention strategies must be built upon this solid foundation of knowledge and a genuine concern for one's group and its members.

A GENERAL MODEL OF INTERVENTION

The first matter at hand is the introduction of a general intervention model relevant to any questions and answers involving group and interpersonal behavior. The model contains five distinct stages; each requires leaders to engage in a process both before and after their actual intervention in the group. These five stages are summarized in Table 13-1.

As the table indicates, the first task facing the leader involves defining the nature and scope of the problem. This entails weaving together theoretical understanding with behavioral observations in order to develop a diagnosis to guide the intervention strategies that will be used. From the more theoretical side, the leader must be sensitive to what we have termed the underlying issues and accompanying consequences that are typically involved in a particular problem. For example, a single member who dominates a discussion can produce an apathetic and nonproductive group as others withdraw their own involvement and let the dominating member carry the ball. The leader must be sensitive to this aspect of the problem.

By observation we simply mean that any intervention in a group must be based upon observational material. Leaders must first observe individual or group behavior, including the patterns of behavior that occur within a group. Their intervention must not only follow from these observations but as importantly must refer back to the behavioral observations. That is, leaders cannot simply intervene like a bolt out of the blue, no matter how exciting, or full of insight their intervention might be. It is hardly helpful for an individual or group members to accept a leader's thoughtful interventions without hearing as well the observational base for those interventions:

> The leader, John, says to a member, Agnes, "I have noticed that you arrive late to most of our meetings. I have also noticed that the group does not begin officially until you arrive. So, when you are very late, as you have often been, we simply wait around, doing little until your arrival. It is getting to be very wasteful of our time. I think this is something we have to examine and do something about."

The diagnostic stage of the intervention process requires that leaders use direct behavioral observations plus their knowledge of theory to make a tentative diagnosis of the problem at hand. A diagnosis is an inference that connects observational material to some larger body of knowledge (e.g., a theory); diagnoses render that material meaningful and direct toward an intervention strategy.

In the preceding example of the late-arriving member, the leader's diagnosis might be that Agnes's late arrival is a power ploy on her part. She knows that the group does not begin until she arrives; she can thereby demonstrate her power and control over he group by managing her arrival time.

Table 13-1. An Intervention Model

DEFINING THE PROBLEM

1. ISSUE:	Why is this a problem?
	What are its dimensions and its possibilities for affecting group process?
2. OBSERVATIONS:	What behaviors do I see taking place within the group and its members?
3. DIAGNOSIS:	What does it mean? What understanding can I conclude about the behavior from my observations and my grasp of the issues that are involved?

ENTERING THE GROUP PROCESS

4. INTERVENTION STRATEGIES:	What are some specific techniques that I can use to enter the group's process to affect the problem?

ASSESSING THE EFFECTS

5. EVALUATION:	What was the effect of my intervention?
	How do I gauge my success or my failure?

It is important to realize that any diagnosis may be incorrect or at best partially correct. Human behavior is determined in a complex multitude of ways. There is no simple, single one-to-one correspondence between a behavior and a given meaning or diagnostic category. Agnes's lateness undoubtedly has other meanings as well: e.g., she had a long way to come to arrive on time for the group meetings. However, when a behavior *becomes consistent over time,* forming a pattern (e.g., her lateness occurs nearly every time the group meets); and when that pattern has a compelling rationale for one meaning over another (e.g., she arrives late even when meetings have been announced well in advance, when she and others have noted meeting times in their notebooks, when leaving in time to make the meeting is possible at least on several occasions); and finally, when other behaviors are noted that form an overall consistency with the diagnosis so that it is not based merely on one action but rather a matrix of behaviors (e.g., the power interpretation is consistent with Agnes's other behavior in the group: she frequently challenges the leader's authority; she seeks to dominate meetings by talking a great deal; she seems to enjoy having members turn to her for advice), then it would appear that the diagnosis is a reasonable one. Basically, as with any diagnostic process, one is looking for multiple operations that converge upon a given diagnosis and make it more compelling than any alternative.

The intervention stage involves the actions that leaders take, what is said and done to effect group process. In Chapter 12 we examined many of these intervention techniques for group leaders. We will pursue these further in this chapter as specific ways to deal with particular issues and problems facing a group.

Evaluation is a necessary follow-up to intervention. The leader's interest is in checking out and evaluating the consequences of his or her intervention. An evaluation can extend from an attempt to validate his or her own analysis against other members' analyses to an effort to judge whether or not the intervention produced the desired effect: e.g., did the group now deal with Agnes's lateness so that members could use their time more effectively together?

Our discussion of the issues that follow will be organized in terms of this model. For each of the seven problems, we will indicate the dimensions or aspects of the problem, the various kinds of observation that are relevant to recognizing it, the kinds of diagnosis that are likely, several useful interventions, and ways to evaluate the effects of these interventions.

DEALING WITH A MEMBER WHO MONOPOLIZES OR DOMINATES THE GROUP

Issue

For most purposes it is desirable for there to be a relative equality of member participation. Most meetings have time limitations; the monopolization of the conversation by any one member deprives others of their fair share of participation. It is useful to think of participation as a resource or commodity within groups. One person who possesses all of that commodity (e.g., by dominating the conversation) denies others their share of this resource. A sense of injustice tends to develop. The issue facing the leader, therefore (or for that matter, members who feel that they are being denied their share of what usually is a scarce resource), is how to deal with this conversational monopolizer.

This is by no means a trivial matter. Several consequences follow from the presence of a monopolizer in a group. The sense of injustice tends to create bad feelings and anger among members; these can be highly disruptive to the group as a whole. Members' anger and frustration may also be directed toward the group's leader, as though asking, "Why don't you do something to stop that person from monopolizing the discussion!" Thus, leaders who refuse to intervene may find themselves a target of group anger, some of it displaced onto them from the more direct target (the monopolizer) and some more directly concerned with his or her failure to handle this type of disruption. Furthermore, if one person dominates the discussion, the kinds of diversity of viewpoint necessary to make group work effective cannot be realized. There are many important reasons, therefore, for the group leader's intervention.

Observations

One does not need a chart and stopwatch in order to observe some of the behavioral manifestations of monopolization. Some things to look for include: incessant talking, almost compulsive in nature; inability to keep still and to listen; tendency to interrupt others who start to talk; tendency to finish others' thoughts and sentences; frequently tangential and confusing style of talking; a driven quality in which what is said is less important than the sheer fact of saying something. Restlessness and inattentiveness among other group members can also be seen as their response to the monopolizer's domination. Symptoms of frustration and anger, especially deflected toward the leader, can usually be noted among the members.

Diagnosis

At one level of analysis, the compulsive, driven quality of talking may reflect a high level of anxiety. If this diagnosis is tentatively made, then other symptoms of anxiety should be sought. For example, does the person fidget, smoke a lot, move about, show excessive body movements?

Excessive talking can also indicate a strong need for attention. A young child may constantly demand parental attention, especially within a competitive setting in which he or she is vying with other children for the favors of the adults. In a group, the monopolizer may be competing with other group members for the attention, recognition, and approval of the leader.

It would not be surprising to discover that compulsive talkers who monopolize the group's time are not very aware either of their behavior or its consequences. They are too busy behaving (e.g., talking) to pause and observe what they are doing or what effects it may have. The major concern here is not psychotherapy—thus we do not probe deeply into the whys and wherefores of the monopolist's behavior. Rather, the goal is primarily to effect a reasonable behavior change. Therefore, we would diagnose the problem as one requiring an intervention that helps the person (a) see his or her behavior, (b) see its effects on the group, (c) change the behavior to give others an opportunity to participate as well. This last point is important. Our intervention goal is not to completely shut off such people from participating in the group, but rather only to help moderate their participation.

Although we may personally diagnose the person's issue as involving anxiety or need for recognition and approval, we would typically be more concerned with effecting a change in behavior (i.e., reducing their domination of the group) than in probing these underlying dynamics. Therefore, while it may be helpful to interpret some of these possibilities to the individual, it is more often better simply to direct our efforts toward the behavior and its effects on the group.

Interventions

There are several types of interventions that we can use. All of them require that we first interrupt and get the individual to hear us. A simple and direct interruption that may be sufficient in some cases would be, for example, "Thank you very much Jones; I really hate to cut you off right here, but I feel that it is important for us to hear from everyone here. Perhaps we can return to you after others have had a chance to speak their piece." This type of interruption can and should be given in a supportive manner: e.g., "That is a very interesting and potentially valuable idea; we only have a short time to meet today, however, and I think it best if we move on. Perhaps we can hear others' responses to your ideas."

In the preceding examples, the leader does not make any real effort to help the person see the behavior and its effects on others. If the compulsive monopolizer has been engaging in this kind of behavior for some time (e.g., over several meetings) or if they have not been responsive to a supportive interruption, the leader might then intervene with one or more of the following.

1. *Reflect behavior:* "Jones, we are really having trouble hearing from everyone today because you are taking up so much time talking. I wonder if you are aware of this." It would be reasonable at this point for the leader to solicit feedback regarding Jones' behavior from others in the group: "Does anyone else feel this way?"

2. *Interpretation:* "Jones, I'm not sure that you are aware that you have talked so much of the time today that hardly anyone else has had a chance. I'm not sure just what it means, but perhaps you're feeling a little anxious about something or concerned with how you come across in this group?" This would be offered as a proposal needing testing. The testing would involve checking with other group members to see if they too feel that Jones is talking excessively and what some of their own interpretations are. In all cases, support is given to Jones to further probe and explore some of the reasons for the behavior.

3. *Reflect group feelings:* "Jones, I've noticed that you have been talking a great deal today—so much so, in fact, that few others have been able to participate. I've also noticed myself and maybe many others in the group are getting bored and frustrated, so I finally stopped hearing what you want to tell us. I really do want to hear what you have to say, but you seem to say so much that I just cannot keep up with it." This also should be followed by checking with others in the group to see if the feelings are shared or are peculiar to the leader.

Even if they are peculiar to the leader, they warrant examination by Jones and the leader.

4. *Confrontation—Individual:* "Jones—could you please shut up for a few minutes? We just aren't getting anywhere, and I really think it would be helpful if you'd be quiet and let a few other people have the floor." This kind of direct confrontation must be carried out in a generally supportive way. A mean or harsh statement may only press everyone into silence and thus not accomplish anything beneficial.

5. *Confrontation—Group:* "I think you should stop talking for a moment; I have something important to ask the others in this group. I've observed that Jones talks a great deal in this group; in fact, so much that none of the rest of you have any opportunity to participate. What I was wondering, however, is why you all have permitted Jones to monopolize the discussion?" This focus on the group's responsibility could also be coupled with an interpretation: "It may be that you all do not want to take any responsibility for working in this group and so eagerly permit Jones to monopolize the discussion."

This last possibility is an important one, especially when we retain our system's perspective on group process. In this view, we must recognize that the other group members may be supporting the domination by one member in order to avoid accepting their own responsibility for their group. The monopolizer, therefore, gets away with the domination but only because other members permit or even want it to be that way. By confronting the group with its behavior, the leader tries to focus on the total field within which the behavior occurs rather than locating the "blame" or full responsibility on the shoulders of the dominating individual.

Evaluation

Almost every intervention presented here is in the form of an open invitation for the individual or for the group to further explore and examine their behavior and its effects. If the invitation is not taken up by the individual or the members, then the leader must reevaluate the intervention approach. The leader may decide, for example, to probe the issue further, to offer additional interpretations or analyses, or perhaps to offer advice regarding a way of improving the equality of participation. A longer-term evaluation depends upon the extent to which the monopolizer stops monopolizing and the other group members take on more responsibility for handling their own participation.

DEALING WITH SILENCE AND APATHY

Issue

If one extreme of member participation involves the monopolizer, the other side involves the silent or apathetic member. The issue, here, however, is more complex. Silence and apathy may describe the behavior of the entire group. In either case, apathy and nonparticipation are some of the most typical and usually frustrating issues for a group's leader.

A few silent members may seem reasonable to the typical leader; yet one of the goals of leadership is to involve all members in the group. This calls for creating a climate within which the silent member feels secure enough to participate. A silent or apathetic group, on the other hand, rarely seems reasonable to any leader; it places the entire burden of responsibility and action on the shoulders of the leader and is not a desirable state of affairs. The leader's goal, therefore, is to understand the basis for several members' or the group's silence and low level of participation and then to intervene in ways designed to increase member involvement. Leaders who carry on soliloquies soon discover that not only are they doing all the work, but the important decisions are not carried out by the very persons who are expected to do this. An involved and actively participating membership is therefore an important goal to achieve.

Silence and apathy of either an individual or the group as a whole can have several different meanings. It is important for the leader to be sensitive to the range of meanings that are possible. Let us begin with an obvious but often ignored possibility. Silence and low participation for the group as a whole may be a direct result of the leader's own style of leadership. That is, silence may be a membership response to an autocratic leadership style. The classroom teacher, for example, who always lectures and dominates the entire class, should not be so puzzled when no one responds to the request, "Are there any questions?" Similarly, leaders who make most decisions for their group in a unilateral manner, who dominate the discussion, who cut off members from participating, and in other ways suggest that this is their group—that they are in charge, and that no one else counts as much as they do—should not be surprised to find member apathy and silence as the typical response. Thus, one of the first things to be examined when a leader encounters general groupwide apathy, nonparticipation, and silence is the leader's own style of leadership.

But silence also conveys other meanings as well. Borrowing from the discussion of Bradford, Stock, and Horwitz (1961), we can outline several reasons for general group silence and apathy:

1. The task facing the group does not seem important to members, even though it may seem important to the leader or to someone external to the group. For example, a health team may be confronted by an outside agency with an issue that members personally do not feel

is particularly relevant. Their silence and general apathy reflects their attitude toward this particular task. Likewise, the leader may impose a task that he or she feels is critical to the group, but fails to inform or persuade others of its critical nature; thus general apathy reflects disinterest in what appears to be an irrelevant task. We are reminded here of a group of medical residents in Family Practice who were discussing various cases; the leader felt that the important task before this group was not simply to discuss a given case, but to examine the implications of members' disagreements concerning the case for their relationships to one another in the group. Members, however, did not see this interpersonal issue as relevant and so resisted the leader's efforts to get them to focus on this issue. Their resistance in this instance took the form of long silences and general disinterest in the entire discussion.

2. The group may feel frustrated if the task or issue seems beyond their present capabilities to handle. In this case, silence and apathy reflect the group's general frustration over its inadequacy to solve a particular problem.

3. Members sense that the issues they must face are frightening or threatening to the group as a whole or to a significant number of them, and so silence becomes a way of avoiding the threatening tasks. To return to the medical residents, it may have been that their silence was a result of their fear of examining their interpersonal relationships. That is, they did not simply define such a discussion as trivial and irrelevant to their major purposes but sensed that to engage in an examination of their own relationships would be too threatening and fearful; their silence and general nonresponsiveness reflected their avoidance of the threat. Recall Bion's concept of *flight* from Chapter 8; flight from a potentially controversial or frightening issue often takes the form of withdrawal into silence and apathy.

4. Silence and apathy, however, are also vehicles that convey the meaning of fight, conflict, and anger. A group may become silent and nonresponsive as a way of dealing with its angry feelings or its internal conflicts. For example, a group may be dominated by a few argumentative members. Other group members may shy away from this form of participation; their silence reflects their inability to deal with the conflict, their fear of getting caught in the battle, or their anger over the dominance and fighting. In other cases, anger toward the leader may take the form of a withdrawal into silence. Much like the pouting child, a group or individual may likewise withhold participation as a way of expressing anger.

Most of the meanings of silence and apathy for the group as a whole can be applied to individual members as well. Thus extremely silent members may be frightened of the topic; may be angry at the leader, the group, or some of its members; may feel that the entire task before then is irrelevant and not properly suited to their purposes; and so forth. Needless to say, silence and apathy are important symptoms of underlying issues facing the individual or the group. It is important for the leader to work toward a diagnosis and intervention before the underlying problems destroy the effectiveness of the group or the contribution of the nonparticipating member(s).

Observation

On the face of it, silence and apathy would appear to be readily observable. Look around the room and spot persons whose participation seems low: they speak infrequently or not at all; they speak only when a direct question is asked of them; they do not respond when a general request for questions is made. There are many further manifestations of silence and apathy that can be observed. These include the following symptoms:

1.   People appear to be bored or disinterested; they yawn, look around the room frequently, seem engaged in other activities than the task at hand, even doze or daydream.

2.   The discussion seems to ramble on; members are unable to keep track of what they are talking about or why.

3.   Few members actively contribute to the group's discussion or work; the burden falls on a few shoulders.

4.   Members arrive late to meetings or absences seem unusually high; members leave early or excuse themselves frequently to leave for other more pressing matters.

5.   Members seem more eager to set the time for the session to end than to deal with the present session itself; there is frequent checking of the time and watches; there is a high level of responsiveness and alertness only when the issues of closing the meeting comes up.

Diagnosis

We have already indicated several meanings that silence and apathy convey. The task of the leader is to make a careful assessment of the specific circumstances at hand in order to sharpen the diagnosis that is made. As we have suggested, apathy and silence can be a reflection of three related matters: leadership style, task issues, and interpersonal issues. Each of these provides a helpful clue to guide the leader's diagnostic search. For example, the leader must first carefully examine his or her own leadership style before jumping to other conclusions regarding the meaning of silence. This means that leaders must be able to process their own behavior (see Chapter 12). Although this is by no means an easy task, it is essential that leaders recognize that they are participants in the group as well as leaders; they can be significant determinants of whatever behavioral effects are observed. It should be obvious that a diagnosis that suggests that the silence and apathy are in response to the leader's style would require an intervention directed toward oneself.

The immediate circumstances surrounding the occurrence of silence provides additional material on which to base the diagnosis regarding its meaning. For example, if the group members have been generally responsive and generally equal in their participation but then suddenly become silent and withdrawn, leaders must ask themselves about the topic or issue that immediately preceded the silence. The discovery may be something as simple as noting, for example, that a conflict between two prominent members of the group has been uncovered; silence may reflect a fearful withdrawal from tampering with this conflict.

To take another example, the leader may have made an intervention that was followed by a silence. In checking out the intervention, the leader may note (as in an earlier example) that members were pushed into a topic or discussion that they felt was either irrelevant or too threatening to pursue. In either case, silence was their response.

Silence, especially of an individual member, does not always reflect a response to something in the immediately present setting; it may reflect some past wound within the group's or individual's life in general. For example, in a group's early meetings, one member may have expressed her views quite openly and forcefully. If the group's response to this member was derisive laughter followed by some rather strong and angry rejections ("That's a stupid thing to say; I thought you knew better than that. Where did you get your training?") the member may become silent in subsequent sessions. Having been wounded once in the group, she fears to move out publicly to express herself again.

Members' past experiences are also reflected in their ongoing group behavior. An individual who is relatively insecure and not confident about himself or his views may be generally silent in group settings. Nothing specific has happened in this group to motivate this behavior; rather the silence reveals something external to the group that leads this person to be a minimal participant.

Interventions

As we have suggested throughout this discussion, the type of intervention that is attempted will depend on the nature of the diagnosis that is made. If leaders suspect that their own style of leadership is the major contributor to members' silence and apathy, then they not only must intervene to change themselves—they also must intervene by helping the group to work through and change its relationships with them. Specifically, leaders will have to check out their analysis against group members' own impressions: e.g., "I've noticed that there is a generally low rate of participation and involvement in this group. I was wondering if you are responding to the way I'm doing things.

Is that contributing to your silence and apathy?"

Unfortunately, there is no magic in handling interpersonal relations; thus a leader who has dominated the group and led autocratically and then suddenly appears to be changing stripes may receive a noncommittal, silent response to a question about leadership style. However, leaders who diagnose their own style as a major contributor to the group's silence must both work actively to change that style and also bring this possibility to the attention of the group. Intervention must be made at two separate but related points: the leader's own behavior and at the group level. The former involves leaders' effort to change their own behavior; the latter involves inviting the group members to respond to the leadership style (e.g., "How is my mode of leadership affecting this group?") and to help negotiate a different style, one that is more conducive to the members' involvement and participation.

Other interventions follow from the diagnosis of the meaning of silence and apathy. For example, the leader may suspect that the group is apathetic because the members think the task before them is not relevant or important. The leader can intervene by suggesting: "I've noticed that there is a general boredom with today's discussion. I wonder if people here feel that what we are doing is not really relevant?" This must be followed up with additional efforts to explore members' feelings about what they are doing and what they would like to be doing: 'How do you feel about today's group? Are there things that you would prefer us to be doing or talking about?'

If leaders sense that the problem facing the group is members' feelings of inadequacy regarding their task, they can intervene by confronting that possibility: "I sense that people don't feel up to handling the issue we are dealing with. Is this generally the way people here feel?" Or leaders may sense that the group's inadequacy stems from lack of structure and organization; they can then intervene to facilitate the development of that structure: "I think that we've all been fumbling about for some time now, not really sure of what to do or how to go about dealing with the problem we're facing. I think it may be helpful if we can develop an agenda of important issues that we must deal with. That is, it may be helpful if we break the larger problem down into smaller parts and tackle each part one at a time. We may find this less frustrating."

If the diagnosis is of silence based on an interpersonal issue, such as fear, anger, or some related emotion, then the leader must decide either to intervene by offering an interpretation ("I wonder if people here are angry at what I've done?" "I wonder if we are afraid to bring up that topic because it may bring bad feelings out into the open") or decide not to intervene, but simply to let the silence pass. This latter approach has much merit, especially when the group has otherwise been moving along well and functioning effectively together. In this case it might take the group too far afield to begin to probe the underlying meanings and bases of the silence when it may just be a passing matter that is better left untouched, given the other purposes and agenda items of the group.

In many groups, an individual's silence should be left alone and untouched; the purpose of the group may not be best served by an attempt to make the group comfortable for a member if such an effort would require the use of too much group time and energy. In the end, it becomes a matter for careful judgment. Leaders must assess the meanings of silence and apathy and the general purposes of the group; they must then judge whether those purposes can be served by declining to intervene in any particular case. Silence, especially of one or a few individuals or as a passing matter within a group, may sometimes be handled best by nonintervention.

Continued silence and apathy, however, are another matter; these must be dealt with actively by the leader.

Evaluation

A successful intervention should be followed by the group's or an individual's overcoming the silence, working through the issue that motivated it, and continuing to function again. One of the best outcomes possible, of course, is that group members become better able to monitor their own behavior and facilitate their own process. In this case, members help one another break free from their silence; members take on increasing responsibility for their own actions and the success or failure of their group; members begin to examine, evaluate, and intervene in their own process—they begin to make their own interpretations of their silences and shorten what otherwise could be a lengthy and time-consuming process. For example, members may realize that when they are silent it means they may be shying away from an important issue that is threating; thus, they quickly try to identify that issue so that they can work more directly and immediately to restore full participation and involvement in their group. Successful interventions, therefore, do not only deal with the short-term issue of silence and apathy but also lay the groundwork for the group to use its own resources to deal with apathy or silence whenever it appears.

DEALING WITH EMOTIONAL OUTBURSTS

Issue

It is the rare group that is formed with the specific task or purpose of encouraging emotional outbursts such as anger and crying. Most groups with which the health professional is involved tend to have cooler norms: members adopt a view that is not hospitable to any excessive display of emotions. Even groups that are formed with the purpose of exploring members' personal experiences and feelings tend to be fearful of any real emotional display. Talking about emotions and feelings may be approved; "doing" the emotions, however, tends to be something of which most disapprove. That group norms tend to forbid or disapprove of actual emotional displays, however, does not mean that emotional outbursts will be absent. Feelings can and often do run high. Anger between members may suddenly break out; or a member may be touched by something that is taking place and begin to cry.

Given the high probability that most groups do not approve of emotional outbursts, the likely response when one occurs is silence, withdrawal, and avoidance. The leader then faces a member who has suddenly let loose a strong feeling and a group that fails to deal with it except by denying its existence. The task for the leader is to intervene helpfully for both.

There are really two related issues. The first involves helping the individual deal with the feelings that have been expressed and with the likely embarrassment over having lost control in a setting that may be inhospitable and nonsupportive. The second involves helping the group develop a more responsible and less avoiding attitude toward such occurrences as well as to explore, where appropriate, the meaning and implication of the outburst in relation to the group's own functioning. This latter point can be especially important for the leader to work with.

In many instances, it is useful to think of the emotionally expressive member as a barometer of the entire group's climate. That person's outburst may be indicative of some underlying tensions within the group as a whole. The individual has lost control and openly expressed what many others might be feeling and experiencing. If this is the case, then the leader must make a special effort to relate the member's outburst to more generally shared group issues. The outburst can thereby become a valuable and important learning experience for the entire group. It is not simply that one member for some mysterious reason has lost control; rather, one member (perhaps with less control than others, a lower boiling point) has openly given vent to feelings that others may also be experiencing.

The two most common emotional displays in groups involve anger and crying. An open display of sexual feelings (e.g., kissing), while a possibility that would likewise have to be dealt with, seems less typical than the other two expressions. We will concentrate our discussion, therefore, around anger and crying. The techniques, however, are applicable whatever form the particular outburst may take.

Observations

Anger can be a very subtle as well as a very direct pattern of behaviors. A true outburst of anger is not difficult to observe: a loud, shouting voice, flushed face, tremors, body postures indicative of fighting. Fists may be clenched; short, choppy movements may be made; speech may be disjointed with a rapid rush of words. Cooler forms of the angry outburst may involve a person who is bordering on a complete loss of control and so seems intent on self-containment: the person may become rigid, leaning forward as though to lunge, yet getting white hands from holding on so tightly to retain control.

In similar manner, crying can range from a readily observed outburst of tears to a more subtle form. In the latter case, one can usually observe tears welling up in the person's eyes; the head is cast downward; they may wring their hands; their lips may tremble; they may withdraw or try to—e.g., cover the face, turn away from the group.

Diagnosis

The diagnostic issue involves an attempt to understand the basis for the member's outburst and also to locate similar feelings within other members of the group. The angry outburst, for example, can represent extreme frustration with what is going on in the group. It can also represent intense disagreement and conflict between members. For some, an angry outburst could represent a way of grabbing for attention. It also often represents "the last straw," reflecting a buildup of unexpressed feelings that finally reach a breaking point. In this instance, the precipitating event may be relatively minor; we must probe into past events in order to understand the intensity of the present response.

Anger, of course, generates anger. Thus, an outburst from one member may be the end point of an escalating cycle that has been building up within the group: i.e., Fred is humorously sarcastic to Bob, who replies with an intense angry comment to Fred who responds with a still more intense jibe at Bob, who finally breaks loose with an angry tirade that embarrasses and silences everyone.

Crying can occur when one member hears something within the discussion that taps some deep-lying feeling within them: e.g., a nurse whose father has recently died suddenly bursts into tears when the group begins to discuss a patient's death. Crying can also represent anger. This may seem paradoxical, but some who consider that the open expression of anger may be inappropriate begin to cry when they are furious. Crying also occurs when people are so overwhelmed by what they are experiencing that they have no behavioral options other than to cry.

Crying when one is happy is another well known possibility. Some psychoanalytically oriented theorists (e.g., Weiss, 1952) have suggested that people cry finally when they feel secure enough to let those feelings emerge into their consciousness. This kind of "crying at the happy ending" suggests that only when we have been reassured that the ending is happy can we permit ourselves to have the sad and tender feelings that we otherwise blocked out. Thus, we may diagnose some crying as indicative of the person's having reached a point of greater security with the group; they finally feel comfortable enough to let themselves cry.

Given the wide range of meanings that can be represented by anger or crying, one of the first tasks facing the leader is to determine what the outburst represents for the member. The intervention strategies, therefore, must include ways to further explore the meanings of such outbursts even while helping support the individual member and helping the group examine the relevance of the outburst to their own functioning.

Interventions

Diagnostic interventions are designed to help the leader and others gain a better sense of the meaning of an outburst; *supportive interventions* are designed to help the member, who may feel embarrassed by the behavior, to deal with the follow-up residues of their outburst. *Group-centered interventions* are designed to help the group members explore both their feelings about what has occurred and the degree to which they too share some of the member's feelings and experiences (i.e., the more general implications of the outburst for the group as a whole).

To help clarify the meaning of the outburst, the leader has several intervention possibilities. The leader may immediately reflect the feelings: "You sound (look) very angry." The leader may provide support in order to help the member clarify the meaning of their outburst:"You must really be upset; let's talk about it." Support and clarification may take the form of saying, for example, "I want you to know that I see your pain and I would like to help. "The leader would then pause, using this intervention as an invitation for the member to continue.

If the nature of the outburst has been extreme—for example, anger that is more than verbal, in fact is overtly physical, or crying that is heading into an hysterical loss of control—one of the first tasks facing the leader is to restore some degree of control. This often requires some actual physical intervention: e.g., getting up and restraining the angry person or embracing the crying person. These are also supportive gestures; they help the person regain some of the lost control, so that they can join in the process of clarification.

Diagnostic interventions can also follow from the leader's interpretations and analyses of the likely meaning of the emotional outburst. These would take the form of testing the leader's analyses rather than being declarations of fact: "You began to cry when we started talking about death. Has there been a recent loss in your own life?" "Your anger at Marge seems out of proportion to what she actually said to you; I wonder if it's got something to do with your attitude toward women?"

It is important for the leader to be supportive while seeking to gain clarification. Likewise, it is important for the leader to invite and encourage the member to examine what has taken place; the leader should avoid pushing, leaving no way out but further retreat into emotional display: "Is this something that you can talk about now?" If the member indicates that he would prefer to wait a while (until some composure is regained), it is then important for the leader to open the invitation again later. That is, the leader should check back with the member and not abandon him after having invited him to examine the situation. This will also help the group members develop increased trust in one another and the ability to be secure in their expressions.

Assuming that the leader has been able to provide support and encouragement for the member and helped her clarify for herself and others the bases of the outburst, it is important for the leader to bring the experience back to the group-centered focus. Recall that the individual member's outburst may reflect sensitivity to an issue that is more generally shared. To test this out the leader can ask the group members directly to get in touch with their own feelings and to share them within the group:

> A group of parents of handicapped children is discussing the difficulties they are experiencing, when suddenly one member begins to cry. The leader helps support that member while encouraging her to explore her crying. The member speaks about her feelings of personal guilt and responsibility for having caused her child's handicap. The leader suspects that this one member's feelings are not unique but are more general to the entire group. Thus, the leader invites the other parents to explore their own feelings, asking, "How do some of the rest of you feel about this?"

By inviting the group members to explore their own feelings, the leader facilitates the involvement of others who may have wished to do this; the leader also helps reduce the distance and separation between the group as a whole and the particular member who had the emotional outburst; all of this, in turn, can help increase the sense of cohesiveness within the group, as members share experiences they might not otherwise have been able to share.

Evaluation

The evaluative issue involves the degree to which the leader's interventions have successfully managed the outburst. In the context we have been discussing, successful management involves at least three related issues: supporting the members who have engaged in the outburst; clarifying the meaning of the outburst; helping the group to examine its own feelings about the outburst and the issues that it represents to members of the group. Successful interventions will be reflected in any or all of the following ways:

—Increased sense of cohesiveness within the group

—Greater openness and willingness to share and talk about feelings

—Integration of the member into the group rather than his or her separation or complete withdrawal

—Ability of the group to face up to difficult matters as they occur rather than to shelve them until they arise later, perhaps with excessive intensity.

Successful interventions, rather than increasing emotional outbursts within a group, should in the long run actually decrease their occurrence. Many outbursts are excessive and disruptive because they occur after a lengthy buildup of tension that is not dealt with when it occurs (this is especially true of anger and frustration). As the leader creates a climate within which members can more openly examine their feelings, the leader will facilitate the development of mechanisms within the group that make future outbursts less likely and less disruptive.

DEALING WITH CONFLICT WITHIN THE GROUP

Issue

As a careful reading of the theories of group development suggests (Chapter 6), conflict is a normal stage in the life of most groups. It is not something, therefore, that by its very nature is bad or destructive; in fact, conflict is often indicative of liveliness and innovation in problem-solving. This being the case, leaders should not uncritically set about to eliminate all conflict that arises within their group; the task, rather, should be to encourage the kind of conflict that can help the group to grow. The constructive use of conflict can become a vital resource to a group.

Having said that, we must also recognize that, carried to an extreme, conflict in the form of bickering, disagreements, nastiness, a tense atmosphere, and such can be more of a hindrance than a helpful resource for a group. It is important to be able to achieve the delicate balance between those conflicts that lead a group astray or into more difficulty and those conflicts that facilitate growth and innovative problem-solving. The task for the leader is to be able to separate destructive conflict from its more constructive form and to help create a climate within which disagreements are dealt with in a reasonable and constructive manner.

There are some useful ways to evaluate whether a conflict is more destructive than helpful (from Bradford, Stock, and Horwitz, 1961):

1. When a group is faced with what appears to be an impossible task, members' frustration over their inability to handle it may erupt in conflict within the group. Such conflict is more an expression of frustration and tension than of the kinds of substantive disagreements that are constructive. It is important for the leader, therefore, to evaluate whether the basis for the conflict within the group is frustration and tension rather than actual disagreements over policies, values, solutions, priorities, and so forth.

2. It is not unusual for members of many groups to be primarily concerned with their personal, individual tasks, especially those involving their own rank and status within the group or within the larger organization in which the group is located. In such cases, members may engage in disagreements and fights as vehicles for expressing or gaining status. Power struggles between individuals, each of whom is attempting to gain the center stage for themselves, or members who talk mainly as a way of being heard by their superiors, typically produce conflicts within a group that are less than constructive.

3. Members may argue and disagree within the group as a reflection of their competing loyalties to outside groups. That is, the group may be composed of individuals who represent different outside groups. The issues that are raised within the group and the conflicts that occur thereby reflect these competing outside loyalties. These conflicts can often prove constructive, especially when the leader can help members relate their inside behavior to these external interests and loyalties and guide them toward some compromise functioning within the group.

4. Conflicts often arise within groups among persons who are all highly invested in the group and its work and who genuinely disagree about procedures, priorities, policies, interpretations, and so forth. These are the kinds of conflicts that can usually prove to be constructive rather than destructive. There are numerous reasons for members to have conflicts with others; when these conflicts are based on highly committed members' genuine differences in point of view and values, then the group can build upon these differences to develop unique, innovative solutions to problems and issues.

Observations

Bradford, Stock, and Horwitz (1961) provide us with some useful symptoms of the various types of conflict that are common within groups. In our previous listing, two bases of conflict were relatively nonproductive (frustration over the task and individual status and power expressions), whereas two other bases were potentially productive (outside loyalties and genuine differences in perspectives and values). The leader who would hope to make a preliminary diagnosis that differentiates between the nonproductive and the productive types will find the following observations helpful:

Some indications that the conflict is *nonproductively* based:

—Every time a suggestion is put forth, it is rejected as being too impractical or impossible.

—Members seem never to have enough time for the group and its tasks and get angry and impatient with one another.

—Members have little sense of what their group is all about, why it exists, what its functions are, and so forth; they are always confused and puzzled.

—Every time an idea is expressed, it is attacked and put down even before it gets fully developed or examined.

—Members line up quickly on one side or another and refuse to negotiate or compromise.

—Members engage in direct or subtle personal attacks on one another.

—The same issues and problems are continually repeated; no solutions are ever found or accepted.

—Members act in ways to win their point or avoid losing their point, showing little concern for or recognition of others or of the group.

—Much talk is self-centered; members seem to participate only when they can be at the center of the group's focus.

Some indications that the conflict is potentially *productive*:

—Members have a goal in mind that they generally agree on and are working toward.

—Members' comments are directed toward the task at hand.

—Members are generally receptive to listening to and hearing others, even though they may respond with disagreement and alternative points of view.

—Members encourage one another to participate, even those with differing points of view.

—Solutions to problems and issues are reached by rational discussion and compromise, and when reached tend not to recur again and again.

—The basis for members' disagreements are openly examined and critically evaluated.

The leader's observations of conflict must attempt to locate both the who and the what of the conflict. The leader must be sensitive to the participants who are involved and what the basis of their conflict is. The particular intervention strategy that is chosen will depend on the diagnosis that is made.

Diagnosis

As we noted, conflict can be built on a potentially productive or a potentially nonproductive base. In the former, the leader uses his or her observations to infer beneficial conflict and intervenes in ways to help the group negotiate these conflicts. In the latter, when the leader infers destructive conflict, working through may not be as useful as some more avoiding approach. There is some indication, for example, that when conflicts are potentially destructive, they should be avoided or played down rather than directly confronted. It becomes a matter for careful judgment and testing out, however.

The leader may sense, for example, that the basis of a conflict between two members involves each member's grab for power and status within the group. The leader recognizes this to be a nonproductive basis for conflict for the group as a whole; the decision is to ignore it and to direct the group away from getting caught up in such a personal struggle. On the other hand, the leader may judge it to be more beneficial for the group to face this issue directly; the decision is to intervene and call the group's attention to what appears to be taking place: "I feel that Smith and Jones are each trying to gain some points in this discussion, and I don't think this is helping us deal with the particular case we are working on. I wonder if you two could either cool it for awhile or let us all explore your behavior with you."

Interventions

Whatever intervention strategy the leader may employ, it is wise to intervene early rather than late. The earlier leaders are able to determine that conflict is present, the earlier they can intervene in the process; early intervention helps thwart an escalating cycle of unproductive conflict. In addition, early intervention that effectively negotiates a resolution to the conflict helps build a firm foundation for using constructive conflicts as a group resource. The group that sees that conflict can occur without tearing the group apart or taking the group too far from its immediate tasks will learn to voice and use conflict and disagreement rather than to shy fearfully away from any open expression of differences.

As with most leader interventions, those involving conflict are also most effective if they occur within a climate of cohesion and trust. A group of individuals who care little for one another or for their group as a whole, who have little trust in anyone including the leader, is not likely to be responsive to most types of conflict-handling interventions. Under such circumstances, the leader will first have to work to facilitate a trusting and cohesive climate within the group; only then can interventions be helpful. Within this general context, however, we can examine several kinds of intervention strategies that the leader can employ:

Interpretation:

I believe that we are having trouble making a decision in our group because we have some rather definite conflicts between various members. I think that we had better look at those conflicts before we try to do any other kinds of work here.

Reflect Behavior:

I've noticed that several members have been silent for quite some time now, that several others are talking a great deal but usually at cross-purposes, that we seem generally unable to keep ourselves focused on anything but fighting and disagreeing.

Reflect Feeling:

I'm not sure how the rest of you feel, but I'm getting annoyed and frustrated over the constant disagreement and bickering that is taking place. I think we have a job to do, and I'd like to get on with it.

Confrontation:

Ms. Carlton, I think you are angry with your supervisor because you feel that if this procedure is accepted, you will no longer have the kind of access to her that you previously had. You seem to feel that the procedure will distance you too much from your supervisor and put too much burden on you. Is that why you are so impatient and are acting so upset with the rest of us?

Voicing the Unmentionable:
I think that you are afraid of losing some power on your service and that is why you are acting so angrily in here, disagreeing with almost everything that is said, even before you give it a full hearing.

We have mentioned only several possible interventions; each is oriented toward pointing out to the individual and to the group that some kind of conflict is present and is thwarting their effectiveness in working together. As we noted earlier, however, our goal may involve helping a group to avoid facing its conflicts altogether.

Assuming that the goal is to help a group effectively use its conflicts, then the leader's task is not simply to point out that there are disagreements, but to help focus the group on these and on their basis; the next step is to facilitate the negotiation of a compromise. This task can be outlined in three separate steps:

—Support and legitimate disagreement and conflict
—Help clarify the basis and meaning of the conflict
—Help negotiate a compromise.

The initial step may involve something as simple as *supporting the idea and the legitimacy of conflict:* "I think we have several disagreements that are being expressed here and I for one think that's a sign of a healthy group." Supporting disagreement is often necessary: it helps members see that they can disagree and not lose their integrity as individuals; that they can disagree and not have their group dissolve; that disagreement can be a useful resource for their group.

Clarifying the basis of conflict, the second step, requires that the leader helps members focus on the actual basis of their disagreements with one another: "I know that the two of you are arguing, but I'm not sure if I fully understand what you are disagreeing about. Maybe you could each stop for a moment and just indicate what your position is." To take another example, the leader might intervene to provide his or her own clarification: "Mr. Zimmer, did you mean that you disagree with Ms. Alison because you feel that the interests of the family as a group are more important than the interests of the patient as an individual? If that is what you meant, then it seems that you and Ms. Alison disagree over the values that medical practice should attempt to implement. I think this is an issue that many of us may have opinions on and should discuss further."

The third step, *negotiating a compromise,* though by no means an easy matter, requires that the leader first focus members on the substantive bases for conflict. The leader and the members are then in a position to examine solutions that all parties can accept and that build upon those areas in which they overlap in their position. The interventions are designed to help members see what they share in common before they get lost in emphasizing ways in which they differ. Once their commonalities are expressed and examined, it becomes possible to see what avenues for satisfactory compromise between opposing perspectives are possible: "I hear Mr. Zimmer saying that he needs more assistance with his department; and I hear Dr. Samuels saying that he is so overloaded at present that he is not able to give anyone any more time. I also note that you both agree that something has to be done. I wonder if it is possible for us to examine some ways for Dr. Samuels to help out Mr. Zimmer's department while receiving help for his own department's patient overload."

Evaluation

The signs of successful conflict resolution will be noted when

—The same old conflicts do not continually emerge over and over again; real solutions that have some durability are achieved

—Members do not fear to express disagreements or to explore their basis and seek some compromise

—Innovative solutions result

—Group cohesiveness and trust seem high even in the midst of much substantive disagreement

—The group does not remain rooted either to an overidealized "honeymoon" or a constant state of warfare; differences as well as similarities are recognized and openly accepted.

Effective handling of conflict results when group members are better able to tolerate and directly deal with their disagreements. Ineffective handling of conflict results either in members' fearing ever to disagree lest all hell break loose or failing to make any progress because they are so burdened by dissension with which they cannot deal. The successful intervention, therefore, will not eliminate conflict from the group but will help the group to use conflict as a productive resource.

DEALING WITH NORMATIVE DEVIANCE

Issue

As we noted in our discussion in Chapter 5, groups develop norms for the behavior that is expected of members. Deviance can be said to occur when a member or several members violate these norms. The typical group response to deviance includes the application of sanctions (e.g., punishment and rejection) and efforts to restore the deviant to proper behavior within the group. Much time may be spent in these efforts to get the deviant member to shape up and fit the group's normative expectations. This is valuable time that usually could be spent in other endeavors. Thus, from the viewpoint of effectiveness, deviancy within a group can deflect the group from its other, often more important activities.

But more than the group may be affected by deviance. Deviant members tend to be less satisfied with their group experience; they may feel anxious and tense. Because they are less valued and even attacked by other members, their self-esteem suffers. Any benefits that group membership can have tend to be lost upon the deviant who is disenfranchised from group involvement. Deviant members are more likely to terminate their membership, to arrive late, attend poorly, and in other ways disrupt the group and their own participation in it. Finally, research has suggested that deviants tend to be prime candidates for becoming casualties or being harmed by the group (Yalom, 1975; Lieberman, Yalom & Miles, 1973). In other words, the leader's responsibility both to the group and to the individual warrants a serious consideration of the deviant member of the group. The tendency is for both the group as a functioning unit and the deviant as an individual to suffer from deviant behavior.

Deviancy develops as a function of two factors: the particular norms of the group and the degree to which a group is open to tolerating deviation from these norms. A deviant, for example, could be someone who wears his hair long in a group that has short hair-length norms and that is intolerant of any variation from its norms. That same person in a more tolerant group may be a deviant in that the norms still call for short hair, but his deviancy does not disrupt him or the group, and does not lead to his rejection from the group; its higher level of tolerance permits a wide latitude of behaviors and appearances.

Given these two factors, the leader's efforts can be directed toward the deviant member's behavior, toward the group's norms, or toward the group's level of tolerance. For example, the leader can try to help the deviant member fit in better with the group; can try to counsel him out of the present group and into a different group; can help support him in his deviance by giving him a greater feeling of acceptance and belonging. However, the leader can also try to help the group change its norms; can help the group become more tolerant in its norms and sanctions for deviancy; can help the group overcome its need for this particular member to change behavior even while the group does not agree to modify its norms.

Notice that the leader's goals involve helping the group as well as the deviant individual. Notice further that the accomplishment of these goals does not demand the single solution of changing the deviant. Rather, there are several possibilities. Deviancy from group norms is not bad or evil; it has consequences for both group and individual, however, that warrant careful leader judgment and intervention.

Observations

The major observational tasks facing the leader involve both a determination of the group's norms and a determination of the intensity of the effect of normative deviation on the individual and on the group. Members who embody and exemplify a group's norms will tend to be highly valued and turned to frequently for their opinions. Those who deviate from the norms will tend to be rejected and devalued by group members. We know that norms can pertain to almost any aspect of behavior or appearance. However, groups typically develop norms regarding such issues as appropriate conversation, appropriate clothing and mannerisms, an appropriate level of emotional expression, the appropriate way of relating to authority and leaders, appropriate ways of dealing with client populations and task issues.

Although we cannot observe norms directly, they can be inferred from our observations of members' behavior and group reactions. Thus our initial task, the determination of a group's norms, can be based on observing group responses to members. Leaders can ask themselves such questions as

—Who receives negative feedback and what about them evokes this feedback? Negative feedback can involve a direct expression—"How dare you come in here looking like that! Don't you know the proper attire for a nurse?" It can also be much more subtle and indirect, ranging from the way the member is looked at (e.g., with eyes and face saying "How dare you...?), to silence, nonresponsiveness and even nonrecognition of the other (e.g., ignoring the person who deviates as though by failing to notice them or to respond to them, they'll disappear). Indirect expressions of negative feedback can also be noted from the ways in which people fight one another or disagree with one another. Scapegoating often reflects the existence of norms from which a member is deviating.

— Who gets the attention? Attention-getting members can often be used as "observational informants" for determining group norms. What about the person brings them so much of the group's attention?

—Who is turned to for opinions and seems to be valued and respected by the group? Again, one can infer a group's norms by observing persons who are most highly esteemed and valued by the group: e.g., members who, when they speak, are listened to; who command attention; who are turned to for their opinions before the group is willing to continue with its discussion; whose favor and approval is frequently sought.

—How would I, as a leader, feel in this member's shoes in this group?

Leaders can ask themselves about the kinds of behavior that they would feel uncomfortable with in this group and the kinds of behavior that they feel to be appropriate. In other words, leaders use themselves as a guideline to understanding the group's norms.

The second observational task facing the leader involves a determination of how consequential the deviancy is on the individual and on the group. Several observational strategies are useful in this determination:

—Is the group repeatedly focusing its attention on a particular member who seems unable to change in ways to satisfy members?

—Does the group spend an inordinate amount of time talking about Ms. X or about issues that are brought up by Ms. X?

—Does the group forever return to Ms. X, putting all other matters aside?

—Does the presence of Ms. X evoke anger or resentment? Does Ms. X seem to have withdrawn (even physically) and become isolated from others in the group?

—Does Ms. X show signs of tension and anxiety or general discomfort?

Basically, the effects of the deviancy must be determined by observing the amount of time spent by the group in focusing on a given member (too much or too little can indicate trouble with that member) and by the nature of the response of that member: e.g., withdrawal, anxiety, tension.

Diagnosis

The diagnostic task facing the leader involves determining the basis for the member's deviancy and the group's response to it *and* the importance of the deviancy to the member and the group. The former question focuses on the meaning of the deviancy: e.g., Does it reflect specific anger on the part of the member? Is it a symptom of some more general disturbance? Is it a matter of cultural differences among members of the group? Is it a reflection of the group's intolerance?

The latter question focuses on the degree to which the deviant behavior is disruptive to the individual or the group. A diagnosis, for example, that the real problem is a more general disturbance might motivate the leader to try (where feasible) to counsel the deviant member out of the group or to help the group avoid its incessant, time-consuming, and unfruitful focus on the deviant member. A diagnosis of a relatively minor disruption, for example, might motivate the leader simply to leave things alone, letting the matter pass. A diagnosis that suggests that the real problem lies with the group's rigid and intolerant norms might motivate the leader to address the group rather than the deviant member.

Interventions

The particular interventions that a leader uses are a function of understanding the meaning of deviancy and a decision about the appropriate target for the intervention. Thus, the leader may make *deviant-centered interventions* or *group-centered inventions,* or both. The former focuses attention on the deviant member and on the meaning of the deviancy. The latter focuses attention on the group's response to the deviant, the norms the deviant is violating, the importance of those norms to the group, its degree of tolerance, and so forth.

Let us suppose that the leader decides initially at least to implement deviant-centered interventions. The leader can then work to clarify the basis for the member's deviancy: e.g., Does it reflect a persistent personal habit (e.g., nail biting)? Does it reflect rejection of the group? Does it reflect anger directed toward the group? Does it reflect ignorance or insensitivity to the group's norms? Does it reveal some personal psychological conflict or need (e.g., the person's low self-confidence motivates him or her to continually solicit positive feedback from others; this constant solicitation proves annoying to others who value confidence in members and disparage displays of what they see as weakness)? Does it reflect a different cultural or class pattern (e.g., members of a different social class or culture may behave in ways that are appropriate to their own group but that violate the norms of the typical middle-class American culture)?

It is important to realize that the type of intervention chosen will reflect the leader's understanding of the meaning of the deviance for the individual and the group. A few examples will help clarify this issue:

—If the deviance means that the member is angry with the group or with someone in the group then interventions must be directed toward the anger rather than the deviant behavior as such: "I've noticed that you always respond to others in this group with what I feel to be anger or resentment. This response seems to run against the grain of this group—we all seem to have agreed not to openly express our anger to one another—and it also seems to be further alienating you from the group. I think it would be helpful if we could talk some about your angry feelings."

—If the deviance reflects ignorance or insensitivity to the group's norms, then interventions can be directed toward helping the member and the group clarify just what these normative expectations are: "I've noticed that some members are annoyed at others' behaviors, but I'm not sure that we understand why. Perhaps it would be useful for us to look at the kinds of expectations we have for one another."

—If the deviance reflects a different cultural or class pattern, then interventions can be directed toward helping the member and the group learn about these cultural differences: "I think we have a great opportunity here to learn more about ourselves by examining our reactions to Ms. Chin; it seems that some of our reactions stem from our cultural differences. It might be very useful for us to understand these differences."

In more general terms, the intervention goal will usually involve opening up the deviant's behavior to group and self-examination. This may be done by reflective techniques: "Your behavior seems somewhat different than that of others in this group; it also seems to be disturbing to some. Maybe we should talk more about it." Or the leader might reflect feelings that he or she is experiencing or suspects that others in the group are experiencing: "I've noticed that whenever you talk, I get somewhat edgy and annoyed at you, as though you say things that people are not supposed to say in this group; I've also noticed some others in the room getting edgy. I wonder if we are feeling anxious and bothered because you act somewhat differently from the rest of us.

The leader can use supportive intervention to the same ends: "I really like some of the things you say and do in here. I've noticed, however, that you behave differently from many other members of this group and that this difference seems to trouble some people."

The leader may choose, on the other hand, to focus more on the group than on the deviant. In this case, interventions will be designed to help the group attend to the deviant's behavior and to their responses and feelings about it: "I've noticed that Alice's appearance is not generally the same as that of other members in this group and that people here seem to be offended by this. I wonder if this is something that we should all examine further?" Or the leader may more simply ask, "How do the rest of you feel about the way Alice dresses?"

It is very difficult to focus on the deviant without further separating that person from the group. Insofar as her separation poses a real problem for her and for the group, it is incumbent upon the leader to attempt to reintegrate the deviant even while calling attention to her unique status: "I'm concerned that some of us are responding negatively to Alice, and I'm not sure that this is good either for her or for our group. I know that we have many other things to do, but I feel that we must take some time out now to deal with our reactions to Alice."

The implication is that whatever specific intervention is selected, *support* is fundamental to handling any normative deviation. Deviants are rarely in a comfortable position in the group, whatever the basis or meaning of their deviancy. They are already separated from others by virtue of their deviant actions; calling attention to their behavior only further separates them. All intervention goals must build upon a firm foundation of support for the deviant, even when it is necessary to counsel them out of the group, work to help them modify or change their behavior, help the group better understand their reactions to the deviant, and so on.

Evaluation

A successful handling of the deviant will prove beneficial both to the group and to the deviant member. The benefit to the deviant, however, may not be a transformation into a nondeviating member; rather, it may more likely involve a change in which the deviancy is no longer disruptive to the group (e.g., excessively time-consuming) and the deviant member no longer suffers the negative consequences of rejection and alienation from the group. It is against this dual standard that leaders must measure and evaluate their success. If the group cannot extricate itself from a continued fascination and involvement with the deviant or if the deviant shows increasing signs of tension and anxiety, then the leader might well consider acting to help extricate the deviant from the group rather than continue with a membership that is disturbing to all.

These are not easy decisions to make; the goals, however, are sufficiently clear; and the various techniques of intervention must be chosen wisely in the service of these goals.

GETTING A GROUP STARTED

Issue

Place yourself in the position of being in a group that has just formed. What are some of the questions you might have? This will provide a useful clue about some of the important issues that are involved whenever a group is getting started. Three major kinds of questions would appear relevant to consider: questions of *who, what,* and *how.* That is, Who is here? What are we to do? How shall we proceed?

Who is here? If the members of the group all know one another from past contacts and work together, this may not seem to be as an important an issue as it would be in a group in which few persons know one another. Yet even with people who have worked together before, a group that is formed with a purpose that is different from their usual contacts will need to have this question answered.

> A nurse was asked by her church group to lead a group dealing with children's sexuality. She was a regular member of the church, as were the parents with whom she was meeting to develop the program for their children. Although everyone in the room had had many previous contacts with one another, they had never before convened around the topic of sexuality. Thus, one of their opening issues involved such questions as: "Who are these other people?" "Can I trust them when I talk about sexual matters?" "Who is this nurse?"

The example suggests that the "who" question is concerned not only with the other members but also with a group's leader or organizer.

The "who" question also contains the issue of trust: Who in here can I trust? Who can I rely on? Who are my friends and allies? Who are my adversaries? As the example suggests, members may know "who" the others in their group are; after all, they have been together in the same church for many years. But they do not know much about "who" these people are in matters of sexuality (the group's purpose for being organized); they do not know whom they can trust to hear about their own views, to respect what they have to say, to listen with caring and concern for their own worries and issues.

Discovering the variety of meanings to the "who" questions thus becomes an important matter in opening a group. It is rarely sufficient simply to begin without some efforts directed toward these issues. Introductions are an important first step. Other interventions will be examined shortly.

Other important questions also exist at the beginning: Why are we here? What are our goals and purposes? Members are generally not only concerned with who is there, but why they have all been convened—i.e., *what* their purposes are. It is imperative for the leader to realize that although he or she may know the reasons they have convened, the members may either not know this reason or may have other goals and purposes of their own. Thus, an early task in the life of a group must be to focus on goals and purposes—"what we are here to do."

How shall we proceed? Members may know who is there and what the joint purposes are, but need help in defining and clarifying how they shall go about accomplishing their goals. Especially if the leader hopes to facilitate a democratically functioning group, it will be important to begin early to develop this style and help members work within its framework.

Observations

There is much to be observed at the opening or first several meetings of the group. Anticipating that issues of who, what, and how will be salient to members provides the leader with an opportunity to focus on the content of what is being said and especially on what is being implied though not directly said. Early sessions in an ongoing group or in the first part of even a short-term group must be devoted to establishing rapport among members and between members and the leader; a sense of trust must emerge.

The absence of trust or anxiety over trust can appear in several forms. (1) Members may be reluctant to open up and talk directly to one another about what they are feeling or about their opinions. Little sharing takes place. (2) The leader may feel that he or she is the prod, doing much of the talking and much of the work. (3) There may be frequent indirect reference to issues of "trust" ("The hospital administration is simply not to be trusted") that may also be reflections of that same issue existing within the group. (4) Statements that are made may get little or no response from others. It is as though nonresponse is used for self-protection ("If I let you talk without probing and responding, then you'll let me talk uncritically and this makes life much safer"). (5) Topics may ramble without much direction, almost disconnected, as though persons are not yet ready to converse in anything more than a polite or superficial manner.

Frustration over a lack of clarity regarding the goals and purposes of the group (the "what" question) may also be readily observed: (1) Members may appear restless and bored; perhaps few will participate. (2) Direct as well as indirect expressions of confusion may frequently occur ("I'm not sure what I'm expected to say;" "I wish we could get some kind of structure to this session"). (3) Frustration may lead to impatience, irritability, and anger; thus, expressions of any of these may occur in response to a need for clarity over goals and purposes.

Finally, "how" issues may be revealed in several ways: (I) Members may not know how to relate to the leader; they may request (directly or typically indirectly), more leadership, more structure, more direction. (2) Members may not be sure how they should go about dealing with the task they face, what procedures should be used, who should speak, how decisions should be made, and so forth.

Diagnosis

As we have noted, who, what, and how questions are relevant to the early life of most groups. These will crop up in many direct as well as disguised forms; the leader should anticipate their occurrence and be prepared to diagnose group or individual difficulties in their terms. In recognition that groups have phases (see Chapter 6 for further details on stages of group development), the leader should know that orientation and inclusion issues (in the form of who, what, and how questions) predominate early in the life of a group. This provides the leader with a ready framework within which to diagnose many of the problems that are likely to occur early on. In other words, knowing the most likely questions and issues that exist when a group is just getting started will help the leader's diagnosis of the members' often unstated agenda items. Members may not directly confront any of these issues; however, they form a part of the unstated or hidden agenda that leaders can use to guide and inform their specific interventions.

Interventions

Because the three major initial issues involve who, what, and how, the leader's interventions must come directly to grips with each of these questions as they are revealed by members' interactions. In the beginning, the best tactic for the leader to follow is to anticipate these issues and lay the groundwork for handling them even before observing their presence. Rather than waiting to observe signs that the group is concerned with "who" (i.e., trust and inclusion), for example, the leader should direct efforts toward helping the group answer these unasked questions.

Early introduction of members, asking them to say something briefly about themselves is important. It is likewise important for leaders to introduce themselves and inform the group about who they are. Anticipating that "inclusion" issues are important, the leader from the beginning should invite members to join in and to participate: e.g., asking for introductions; inviting feedback and expressions of opinions and points of view.

Trust does not occur magically; it evolves from a context in which members begin to feel secure with one another and with their group leader. The leader can contribute significantly to this sense of security by acting in supportive and encouraging ways. Leaders who open with a fast-fire critique are clearly informing members that they are in a risky situation—beware. Expressions of support for members who begin to participate; inviting members to join in, to share, and to be heard: all of these are helpful early interventions that help establish a sense of rapport and trust. Modeling desirable behavior (e.g., supportive, attentive listening, concern) can likewise be most helpful in early leader interventions.

Questions of "what" (What are our goals and purposes?) must also be dealt with very early. In this too, the leader's ability to anticipate this issue can help short-circuit problems that might otherwise develop. Interventions here should help members focus on their own purposes for the group; likewise, purposes that the leader has or that are given to the group from "external sources" (e.g., hospital administration) must be openly introduced and examined. Much opening work must be devoted to an expression of goals and purposes (members, leaders, organizations), and to a negotiation over the goals and purposes and the priorities of the group.

The leader's interventions must help members develop their own goals, negotiate with others over what the group's goals will be, and set priorities. The latter offers a useful way of organizing what may appear to be diverse sets of goals by locating some of them at the top of the list for immediate consideration and action and others lower down for later consideration and action.

Interventions that are designed to deal with questions of "how" are also necessary for early work. Let us suppose that the leader desires to establish a democratic leadership style, one in which members adopt the following as their own procedures of operation: taking responsibility for their group; working together toward commonly defined goals; negotiating decisions rather than accepting the will of the most dominant member or leader. In this case the leader must intervene with this style from the very beginning.

It is often useful for the leader to inform the group about his or her preferred mode of leading: "I prefer to help facilitate group discussion rather than to lead in the typical manner; thus I see my role as helping members participate, to invite your participation and involvement in the group." It is likewise important for leaders to adopt this style in their mode of interacting in the group: e.g., to invite members participation; to help clarify; to summarize, paraphrase, and reflect; to process the ongoing interaction. Creating a group in which a democratic style exists and in which members take responsibilities for processing and providing feedback to one another about what their group is doing—all this must start with the first session.

Evaluation

A successful beginning is one that deals with the three opening issues that confront all groups: Who is here? What are our goals and purposes? How shall we go about working together? Failure to handle the issue of "who" will lead to low trust and insufficient rapport for the group to work well together. Failure to handle the issue of "what" will lead to high levels of frustration and confusion, withdrawal into apathy, and reluctance to participate further in so ill-defined and disorganized a group. Failure to handle the "how" question will lead to inability to act—that is, an inability either to make decisions or to act upon and implement the decisions that are made. Success, on the other hand, exists when members begin to feel that they know who is there; they develop a sense of reasonable security in participating and in sharing their own views and opinions; they have a sense that they know their purposes and how the group can proceed to handle them and reach their negotiated goals; they feel that their own interests have been merged into the group's purposes and that their needs will be taken care of as the group goes about its business.

TERMINATING A GROUP

Issue

Terminating a group can involve several things: something as simple as the end of one meeting when many others are still planned; the end of a group that has been meeting together for sometime but is now ending; the end of a group that has convened only once or a few times. To end, though it carries a different intensity of feeling in each case, still poses certain issues with which the leader and members must deal. For example:

1. What have we accomplished in our time together?
2. Have our goals been achieved or have we failed?
3. How do we feel about leaving one another? Is there a sense of loss?
4. Is this really the end or just a break? Do we need to continue our group or arrange for additional times together?

Long-term groups or even short-term groups that have developed a strong, close bond face an especially difficult issue in terminating. Terminating in such instances implies *loss;* the usual response to loss is grieving and often anger. If a group has developed close relationship, then on terminating, people anticipate the loss of their group and relationships; even though some individuals may continue to have contact, the group as a living entity will be over. Members may need to grieve over this loss; one important component of that grieving is often a sense of anger: e.g., "You are all abandoning me."

Short-term groups in which no substantial personal bonding has occurred will tend to experience much less loss and less need to grieve; such a group will nevertheless have terminating issues typically involving more task-related matters and matters of personal self-esteem. If the interpersonal bonds have not been intense, then their termination will not be as critical an issue as in those groups in which such bonds have developed. However, task-related issues will be important. In particular, members' self-esteem may be embedded in their group success or failure on their task: "If we failed to reach our goals, am I responsible for that failure?" Thus, termination can mean "failure" or "success," lowered self-esteem or higher self-esteem.

Needless to say, the leader cannot simply come to the end of the life of a group and leave without helping the group deal with its termination issues. This means sufficient time must be allowed for the group to examine those issues (not the last two minutes of the final meeting) and to work through members' feelings about their group and its accomplishments. The leader can anticipate members' denial and avoidance of terminating issues; this means that the leader bears special responsibility to help the group probe the meaning of its termination. The leader, likewise, will have to be able to interpret symptoms of termination: e.g., lateness, apathy, refusal to engage in deep or meaningful discussions, angry, seemingly unfocused feelings, premature termination, and withdrawal. The latter is especially important in that many groups will try to terminate long before their actual end and thus withdraw all their involvement, leaving the last several sessions with no action, no decisions, no caring.

Observations

Knowing that terminating is an important issue, the leader must be prepared to observe early warning signs. As noted, these can include a diverse array of members' behaviors that are linked to terminating. (1) Members who formerly talked rather openly and easily together now may seem to have reverted to modes of defensiveness and superficiality. (2) Anger may seem to be prevalent as though members are upset with their leader or with one another, with no clear or apparent "stimulus" other than the imminent end of the group. (3) Conversation may shift toward discussions of death, dying, failure, loss, or some other such theme that suggests the feelings that termination bring to the forefront. (4) Members may begin to talk about or make plans for meeting beyond the final time; some urge a continuation of the group as if by continuing they can avoid dealing with their feelings of termination. (5) Some members may begin to withdraw, to come late to meetings, to miss meetings, to act as though the group is over and no longer a relevant matter for them.

Diagnosis

We diagnose that the issue is one of termination from a combination of behaviors we observe and our awareness that the time for the group's ending is near. Behavior early in the life of a group that is scheduled for ten meetings means something different from what appears to be that same behavior during the ninth meeting: e.g., talking about loss and grief early in a group may refer to some external issue, whereas that same talk during the ninth meeting may be indicative of concern with this group's own termination and the feelings that are then surfaced.

We have suggested two separable though related diagnoses on what we have termed termination issues: the one focuses on *interpersonal issues* and themes; the other centers on *task-related issues* and themes. Interpersonal issues are very likely whenever group members have established an intense bonding to one another or to the leader. These issues, involving loss, helplessness, vulnerability, grief, and anger, are also especially likely to occur among those members who have shared or disclosed more of themselves in the group. They can feel the loss most keenly or be most angry that "they gave," but there is no longer any time for others to reciprocate. Taking risks and disclosing oneself in a group not only helps cement bonds of trust and caring; it also lays a foundation for often intense feelings of loss on termination.

Task-related termination issues, as we have noted, are concerned especially with feelings of success and failure; basically these are matters of individual self-worth and self-esteem. Having been a member of a group that stated its goals and accomplished them can make termination a positive experience by comparison with a group that failed to reach its goals or produced a product or made decisions that few were pleased with. In the latter case, termination, although it may seem like a relief, can also contain the seeds for self-doubt and lowered self-esteem. Such possibilities are at least worthy of being explored within the group.

Interventions

The primary task of the group leader is to help the group engage its own termination issues, face them, and work them through. This means that the leader must recognize the symptoms of termination and help the group interpret these: "I sense that several of you are very angry that we have only two meetings remaining. I've noticed that people seem to be coming in later and later. Perhaps we are concerned with our termination and should look at how we feel about this." Or the leader might observe that members seem unable to leave any given meeting; they hang around and wait and wait, not wanting to be the first to leave. This too might be interpreted to the group as a termination issue.

The leader's role is to intervene by interpreting behaviors as reflections of termination and by asking the members to probe their feelings about termination. This can often be facilitated by the leader's own sharing. How does he or she feel about this group coming to an end? Leaders' feelings often provide useful clues about members' feelings. If the leader genuinely feels a sense of loss, it is likely that other members will also share this feeling. If the leader feels frustrated and angry at the group for having failed to work well, it is likely that other members will share many of these same feelings. Thus, interventions can be helpfully guided by leaders' analysis of their own feelings on termination.

Knowing that termination themes involve loss as well as self-esteem will help determine the leader's interventions. The leader can directly ask members how they feel about their group's work together. Do they feel a sense of pride in what they have done or a sense of failure? Do they feel themselves responsible for what has taken place or not responsible?

Two critical issues that the leader faces involve either terminating too early or avoidance and denial of termination. In either case, the leader must intervene. The first situation requires interventions that remind members that they still have much time together and that any behavior that appears like termination is not appropriate this early. The latter calls for the leader to confront members with their worries about terminating, interpreting their behavior in these terms, and then help members openly explore and examine their feelings.

Evaluation

Successful termination will leave members with a valid sense of their experience and work together. They will come away not denying their involvement and self-disclosures nor being embarrassed or ashamed, but rather remembering the good times, the good feelings, the caring and concern that they and others shared. A good termination, in other words, will help members as they approach and enter other group experiences. A poor termination can sour members on interpersonal relations; they will come away feeling that they became involved but to no end, to no purpose other than the pain and anger of loss.

Successful termination, even when group members have not worked well together and have basically failed to accomplish the group tasks, will leave members with a knowledge of why they failed and how they can proceed better in their next group or committee involvement. In other words, successful termination will help members learn from their failures as well as enjoy their successes. Leaders must evaluate their own success in handling termination issues in these terms. Their goals will have been accomplished if failure becomes a building block for later success and if self-disclosure and intense bonding becomes a welcome rather than a frightening future prospect.

SUMMARY AND CONCLUSIONS

This chapter has sought to introduce the prospective group leader to some of the major questions that are asked and some of the ways of thinking about and providing answers to those questions. A general intervention model was introduced. This model calls on the leader to undertake a pre-intervention analysis, adopt an intervention strategy based on that analysis, and finally to evaluate the success of the intervention chosen. Pre-intervention questions require the leader to define the nature of the problem or issue. This includes examining why something is a problem, what observations are made, and what diagnosis emerges from an understanding of the nature of the problem and these observations. Intervention strategies vary as a function of the specific diagnosis made; they include the entire range of feedback and processing approaches we have considered in this and other chapters (e.g., Chapter 12). Post-intervention evaluation requires leaders to gauge the success or failure of their analysis and intervention in terms of certain criteria, examined in this chapter.

Whatever the particular intervention approach adopted, effective leadership must build upon four critical elements: genuine care and concern for the group, its members, and its functioning together; knowledge of group process concepts and theories; development of the perceptual and interpersonal skills needed to intervene in a group's ongoing process; sensitivity to oneself and one's impact on group process as a participant-observer. These four factors are like the legs of a table; any one that is missing causes wobbling, uncertainty, insecurity.

This text (and this chapter) has stressed three of these four elements; the fourth—genuine care and concern—while not as readily taught, often derives from the sense of self-confidence that the other three elements provide. As individuals develop a solid foundation in group process concepts and theory, the perceptual and interpersonal skills required to intervene in a group, and awareness of themselves as a participant in the process of the group, they can acquire a greater interest in and concern for the group they lead or in which they are members. It is difficult not to develop this genuine concern once we know something about how groups function and about the ways we can intervene to facilitate the improvement of that functioning.

References

Aday, L.A. (1987). The ethical implications of prospective payment and corporate medical practice: A research agenda. *Social Justice Research, 1.* 275–296.

Allport, G. W. & Odbert, H. S. (1936). Trait names: A psycholexical study. *Psychological Monographs, 47,* no. 211.

Argyle, M. & Dean, J. (1965). Eye contact, distance and affiliation. *Sociometry, 28,* 289-304.

Argyris, C. (1975). Dangers in applying results from experimental social psychology. *American Psychologist, 30,* 469-485.

Argyris, C. (1969). The incompleteness of social psychological theory. *American Psychologist, 24,* 893-908.

Argyris, C. (1976). Theories of action that inhibit individual learning. *American Psychologist, 31,* 638-654.

Argyris, C. & Schon, D. (1974). *Theory in practice.* San Francisco, Ca.: Jossey-Bass.

Asch, S. E. (1952). *Social psychology,* Englewood Cliffs, N.J.: Prentice-Hall.

Axelrod, R. (1984). *The evolution of cooperation.* New York: Basic Books.

Bales, R. F. (1955). Adaptive and integrative changes as sources of strain in social systems. In A.P. Hare, E. F. Borgatta & R. F. Bales (Eds.), *Small groups.* New York: Knopf.

Bales, R. F. (1955). The equilibrium problem in small groups. In A. P Hare, E. F. Borgatta & R. F. Bales (Eds.), *Small groups.* New York: Knopf.

Bales, R. F. (1950a). *Interaction process analysis: A method for the study of small groups.* Reading, Ma: Addison-Wesley.

Bales, R. F. (1950b). A set of categories for the analysis of small group interaction. *American Sociological Review, 15,* 257-263.

Bales, R. F. (1970). *Personality and interpersonal behavior.* New York: Holt, Rinehart & Winston.

Bales, R. F. (1958). Task roles and social roles in problem-solving groups. In E. E. Maccoby, T. M. Newcomb & E. L. Hartley (Eds.), *Readings in social psychology* (3rd Ed.). New York: Holt Rinehart & Winston.

Bass, B. M. (1960). *Leadership, psychology, and organizational behavior.* New York: Harper & Row.

Bateson, G. (1972). *Steps to an ecology of mind.* New York: Ballantine.

Bateson, G., Jackson, D., Haley, J & Weakland, J. (1956). Toward a theory of schizophrenia. *Behavioral science, 1,* 251-264.

Bavelas, A. (1950). Communication patterns in task-oriented groups. *Journal of the Acoustical Society of America, 22,* 725-730.

Bellah, R. N., Madsen, R., Sullivan, W. M. Swidler, A., & Tipton, S. M. (1985). *Habits of the heart: Individualism and commitment in American life.* Berkeley, CA: University of California Press

Benne, K. D. & Sheats, P. (1948). Functional roles of group members. *Journal of Social Issues, 4.*

Bennis, W. B. & Shepard, H. A. (1956). A theory of group development. *Human Relations, 9,* 415-438.

Berger, P. L. & Luckman, T. (1966). *The social construction of reality.* New York: Doubleday.

Berkman, L. F. & Syme, S. L. (1979). Social networks, host resistance, and mortality: A nine-year follow-up study of Alameda County residents. *American Journal of Epidemiology, 109.* 186-204.

Bernstein, B. (1971). *Class, codes, and control, I: Theoretical studies towards a sociology of language.* London: Routledge & Kegan Paul.

Bernstein, B. (Ed.) (1973). *Class, codes and control, II: Applied studies towards a sociology of language.* London: Routledge & Kegan Paul.

Bertalanffy, L. von (1950). An outline of general system theory. *British Journal of a Philosophy of Science, 1,* 134-165.

Biddle, B. J. & Thomas, E. J. (Eds.) (1966). *Role theory: concepts and research.* New York: Wiley.

Billig, M. G. (1976). *Social psychology and intergroup relations.* London: Academic Press.

Bion, W. R. (1959). *Experiences in groups.* New York: Basic Books.

Birdwhistell, R. (1952). *Introduction to kinesics: An annotation system for analysis of body motion and gesture.* Lousiville, KY: University of Louisville Press.

Blom, J. P. & Gumperz, J. J. (1972). Some social determinants of verbal behavior. In J. J. Gumperz and D. Hymes (Eds.), *Directions in sociolinguistics.* New York: Holt Rinehart & Winston.

Borgatta, E. F., Couch, A. S. & Bales, R. F. (1954). Some findings relevant to the great man theory of leadership. *American Sociological Review, 19,* 755-759.

Bowlby, J. (1969). *Attachment and loss, Vol. 1, Attachment.* New York: Basic Books.

Bowlby, J. (1973). *Attachment and loss, Vol. 2, Separation.* New York: Basic Books.

Bradford, L. P. & Lippitt, R. (1961). Building a democratic work group. In G. L. Lippitt (Ed.), *Leadership in action.* Washington, D. C.: National Training Laboratories, National Education Association.

Bradford, L. P., Stock, D. & Horwitz, M. (1961). How to diagnose group problems. In L. Bradford (Ed,), *Group development.* Washington, D. C.: National Training Laboratories, National Education Association.

Brown, R. W. & Ford, M. (1961). Address in American English. *Journal of Abnormal and Social Psychology, 62,* 375-385.

Brown, R. W. & Gilman, A. (1960). The pronouns of power and solidarity. In T. Sebeck (Ed.), *Style in language: Conference on style Indiana University, 1958*. Cambridge, MA: Technology Press of MIT.

Brownell, A. & Shumaker, S. A. (Eds.) (1984). Social support: New perspectives in theory, research, and intervention. Part I. Theory and research. *Journal of Social Issues, 40,* no. 4.

Buck, R., Miller, R. E. & Caul, W. F. (1974). Sex, personality, and physiological variables in the communication of affect via facial expression. *Journal of Personality and Social Psychology, 30,* 587-596.

Buono, A. F., Bowditch, J. L. & Lewis, J. W. (1985). When cultures collide: The anatomy of a merger. *Human Relations, 38,* 477-500.

Carroll, J. S., Bazerman, M. H. & Maury, R. (1988). Negotiator cognitions: A descriptive approach to negotiators' understanding of their opponents. *Organizational Behavior and Human Decision Processes, 4,* 352-370.

Cartwright, D. & Zander, A. (1968). *Group Dynamics* (3rd Ed.). New York: Harper & Row.

Clausen, J. A. (1963). Social factors in disease. *Annals of the American Academy of Political and Social Science, 346,* 138-148.

Cobb, S. (1976). Social support as a moderator of life stress. *Psychosomatic Medicine, 38,* 301-314.

Cohen, R. L. (1987). Distributive justice: Theory and research. *Social Justice Research, 1,* 19-40.

Cohen S. & Wills, T. A. (1985). Stress, social support, and the buffering hypothesis. *Psychological Bulletin, 98,* 310-357.

Cooley, C. H. (1909) *Social organization: A study of the larger mind*. New York: Scribner's.

Croog, S. H. (1961). Ethnic origins, educational level, and responses to a health questionnaire. *Human Organization, 20,* 65-70.

Cumming, J. & Cumming, C. (1962). *Ego and milieu*. New York: Atherton.

Daniels, D. N. & Rubing, R. S. (1968). The community meeting. *Archives of General Psychiatry, 18,* 60-75.

Deutsch, M. (1953). The effects of cooperation and competition upon group processes. In D. Cartwright & A. F. Zander (Eds.), *Group dynamics: Research and theory*. Evanston, IL: Row, Peterson.

Deutsch, M. (1969). Conflicts: Productive and destructive (Kurt Lewin Memorial Address). *Journal of Social Issues, 25,* 7-41.

Deutsch, M. (1962). Cooperation and trust: Some theoretical notes. In M. R. Jones (Ed.), *Nebraska Symposium on Motivation*. Lincoln: University of Nebraska Press.

Deutsch, M. & Gerard, H. B. (1955). A study of normative and informational social influences upon individual judgment. *Journal of Abnormal and Social Psychology, 51,* 629-636.

Deutsch, M., Pepitone, A & Zander, A. (1948). Leadership in the small group. *Journal of Social Issues, 4.*

Dewey, J. & Bentley, A. F. (1949). *Knowing and the known*. Boston: Beacon Press.

Duncan, B. L. (1976). Differenttial social perception and attribution of inter-group violences: Testing the lower limits of stereotyping of blacks. *Journal of Personality and Social Psychology, 34,* 590-598.

Dunkel-Schetter, C. (1984). Social support and cancer: Findings based on patient interviews and their implications. *Journal of Social Issues, 40,* 77-98.

Ekman, P. (1964). Body position, facial expression and verbal behavior during interviews. *Journal of Abnormal and Social Psychology, 68,* 295-301.

Ekman, P. (1965a). Commmunication through non-verbal behavior: A source of information about interpersonal relations. In S. S. Tomkins & C. E. Izard (Eds.), *Affect, cognition, and personality: Empirical studies.* New York: Springer.

Ekman, P. (1965b). Differential communication of affect by head and body cues. *Journal of Personality and Social Psychology, 2, 726-735.*

Ekman, P. & Friesen, W. V. (1974). Detecting deception from the body or face. *Journal of Personality and Social Psychology, 29,* 288-298.

Ekman, P. & Friesen, W. V. (1962). Non-verbal leakage and clues to deception. *Psychiatry, 32,* 88-106.

Ekman, P., Friesen, W. V. & Ellsworth, P. (1972). *Emotion in the human face: Guidelines for research and an integration of findings.* New York: Pergamon Press.

Ellsworth, P. C. & Carlsmith, J. M. (1968). Effects of eye contact and verbal contact on affective responses to a dyadic interaction. *Journal of Personality and Social Psychology, 10,* 15-20.

Emerson, J. (1975). Behavior in private places: Sustaining definitions of reality in gynecological examinations. In D. Brissett & C. Edgley (Eds.), *Life as theater.* Chicago: Aldine.

Ervin-Tripp, S. (1969). Sociolinguistics. In L. Berkowitz (Ed.), *Advances in experimental social psychology.* Vol. 4. New York: Academic.

Exline, R. (1971). Visual interaction: The glances of power and preference. *Nebraska Symposium on motivation, 19,* 163-206.

Festinger, L. (1954). A theory of social comparison processes. *Human Relations, 7,* 117-140.

Festinger, L., Schachter, S. & Back, K. (1950). *Social pressures in informal groups: A study of human factors in housing.* New York: Harper.

Fielder, F. E. (1967). *A theory of leadership effectiveness.* New York: McGraw-Hill.

Fiorelli, J. S. (1988). Power in work groups: Team member's perspectives. *Human Relations, 41,* 1-12.

Firman, G. J. & Kaplan, M. P. (1978). Staff splitting on medical-surgical wards. *Psychiatry, 41,* 289-295.

Freedman, N., Blass, T., Rifkin, A. & Quitkin, F. (1973). Body movements and the verbal encoding of agressive affect. *Journal of Personality and Social Psychology, 26,* 72-85.

French, J. R. P., Jr. & Raven, B. H. (1959). The bases of social power. In D. Cartwright (Ed.), *Studies in social power.* Ann Arbor, MI: Institute for Social Research, University of Michigan.

Gibb, C. A. (1969). Leadership. In G. Lindzey & E. Aronson (Eds.), *Handbook of social psychology* (2nd Ed.). Vol. 4. Reading, MA: Addison-Wesley.

Greenwald, A. G. (1980). The totalitarian ego: Fabrication and revision of personal history. *American Psychologist, 35,* 603-618.

Gumperz, J. J. & Hymes, D. (Eds.). (1972). *Directions in sociolinguistics.* New York: Holt, Rinehart & Winston.

Haber, J., Leach, A. M., Schudy, S. M. & Sideleau, B. F. (1982). *Comprehensive psychiatric nursing,* (2nd Ed.). New York: McGraw-Hill.

Hall, E. T. (1963). Proxemics: The sutdy of man's spatial relations. In I. Galdston (Ed.), *Man's image in medicine and anthropology: Arden House Conference on Medicine and Anthropology, 1961,* New York: International Universities Press.

Hall, E. T. (1959). *The silent language.* Garden City, N.Y.; Doubleday.

Hare, A. P. (1962). *Handbook of small group research.* Glencoe, IL: Free Press

Hare, A. P. (1952). A study of interaction and consensus in different sized groups. *American Sociological Review, 17,* 261-267.

Harlow, H. (1962). The heterosexual affectional system in monkeys. *American Psychologist, 17,* 1-9.

Harm, C. S. & Golden, J. (1961). Group worker's role in guiding social progress in a medical institution. *Social Work, 6,* 44-51.

Heelas, P. & Lock, A. (Eds.). *Indigenous psychologies: The anthropology of the self.* London: Academic Press.

Henley, N. M. (1977). *Body politics: Power, sex, and nonverbal communication.* Englewood Cliffs, N.J.: Prentice-Hall.

Hinrichsen, G. A., Revenson, T. A. & Shinn, M. (1985). Does self-help help? An empirical investigation of scoliosis peer support groups. *Journal of Social Issues, 41,* 65-87.

Hofstede, G. (1980). *Culture's consequences: International differences in work-related values.* Beverly Hills, CA: Sage

Hollander, E. P. (1958). Conformity, status and indiosyncrasy credit. *Psychological Review, 65,* 117-127.

Homans, G. C. (1950) *The Human group.* New York: Harcourt.

Hyman, H. H. (1942). The psychology of status. *Archives of Psychology, 38,* 269.

Hymes, D. (Ed.) (1964). *Language in culture and society: A reader in linguistics and anthropology.* New York: Harper & Row.

Hyrcenko, I. & Minton, H. L. (1974). Internal-external control, power position, and satisfaction in task-oriented groups. *Journal of Personality and Social Psychology, 30,* 871-878.

Ishisaka, H. A., Nguyen, Q. T. & Okimoto, J. T. (1985). The role of culture in the mental health treatment of Indochinese refugees. In T. C. O. Owan (Ed.), *Southeast Asian Mental Helath,* pp. 41-65. U. S. Department of Health and Human Services Publication.

Jackson, J. M. (1959) A space for conceptualizing person-group relationships. *Human Relations, 12,* 3-15.

Janis, I. L. (1973). Groupthink among policy makers. In N. Sanford & C. Comstock (Eds.), *Sanctions for evil*. San Francisco: Jossey-Bass.

Jemmott, J. B. & Magliore, K. (1988). Academic stress, social support, and secretory immunoglobulin A. *Journal of Personality andd Social Psychology, 55*. 803-810.

Jones, E. E. & Gerard, H. B. (1967). *Foundations of social psychology*. New York: Wiley.

Jones, M. (1953). *The therapeutic community*. New York: Basic Books.

Jourard, S. M. (1968). *Disclosing man to himself*. Princeton, N.J.: Van Nostrand.

Kasl, S. V. & Mahl, G. F. (1965). The relationship of disturbances and hesitations in spontaneous speech to anxiety. *Journal of Personality and Social Psychology, 1*, 425-433.

Kelley, H. H. (1973). The processes of causal attribution. *American Psychologist, 28*, 107-128.

Kelley, H. H. & Stahelski, A. J. (1970). Social interaction basis of cooperators' and competitors' beliefs about others. *Journal of Personality and Social Psychology, 16*, 66-91.

Kiesler, C. A. & Morton, T. L. (1988). Psychology and public policy in the "Health care revolution". *American Psychologist, 43*, 993-1003.

Kilmann, R. H. (1985). Corporate culture. *Psychology Today*, April.

Kinzie, J. D. (1985). Overview of clinical issues in the treatment of Southeast Asian refugees. In T. C. O. Owan (Ed.), *Southeast Asian Mental Health*. pp. 113-135. U. S. Department of Health and Human Services Publication.

Klein, M. (1948). *Contributions to psychoanalysis: 1921-1945*. London: Hogarth.

Kramon, G. (January 8, 1989). Taking a scapel to health costs. *New York Times*.

Kressel, K. & Pruitt, D. G. (1985). Themes in the mediation of social conflict. *Journal of Social Issues, 41*, 179-198.

Labov, W. (1972). *Sociolinguistic patterns*. Philadelphia: University of Pennsylvania Press.

Labov, W. (1966). *The social stratification of English in New York City*. Washington, D.C.: Center for Applied Linguistics.

Learmonth, G. J., Ackerly, W. & Kaplan, M. (1959). Relationships between palmar skin potential during stress and personality variables. *Psychosomatic Medicine, 21*, 150-157.

Leavitt, H. J. (1958). Some effects of certain communication patterns on group performance. In E. E. Maccoby, T. M. Newcomb & E. L. Hartley (Eds.), *Readings in social psychology* (3rd Ed.). New York: Holt.

Leiter, M. P. (1988). Burnout as a function of communication patterns: A study of a multidisciplinary mental health team. *Group and Organization Studies, 13*, 111-128.

Lewin, K. (1947a). Frontiers in group dynamics, I: Concept, method and reality in social science: Social equilibria and social change. *Human Relations*, 5-41.

Lewin, K. (1947b). Frontiers in group dynamics, II: Channels of group life; social planning and action research. *Human Relations*, 143-153.

Lewin, K. (1958). Group decision and social change. In E. E. Maccoby, T. M. Newcomb & E. L. Hartley (Eds.), *Readings in social psychology* (3rd Ed.). New York: Holt, Rinehart & Winston.

Lichtman, R. & Wolfe, B. (Eds). (1987). Equity and the allocation of health care resources. *Social Justice Research, 1,* No. 3.

Lieberman, M. A., Yalom, I. D. & Miles, M. B. (1973). *Encounter groups: First facts.* New York: Basic Books.

Linton, R. (1936). *The study of man.* New York: Appleton-Century.

Lippitt, G. L. (1961). How to get results from a group. In L. P. Bradford (Ed.), *Group Development.* Washington, D.C.:National Training Laboratories, National Education Association.

Lippitt, R. & White, R. K. (1958). An experimental study of leadership and group life. In E. E. Maccoby, T. M. Newcomb and E. L. Hartley (Eds.), *Readings in social Psychology* (3rd Ed). New York: Holt, Rinehart & Winston.

Little, K. B. (1968). Cultural variations in social schemata. *Journal of Personality and Social Psychology, 10,* 1-7.

Litwak, E. & Szelenyi, I. Primary group structures and their functions: Kin, neighbors, and friends. *American Sociological Review, 34,* 465-481.

Luft, J. (1970). *Group processes,* (2nd Ed.). Palo Alto, CA: National Press.

Maier, N. R. F. (1970). *Problem solving and creativity in individuals and groups.* Belmont, CA: Brooks/Cole.

Maslach, C. (1978). The client role in staff burnout. *Journal of Social Issues, 34,* 111-124.

McClintock, C. G. & Liebrand, W. B. G. (1988). Role of interdependence structure, individual value orientation, and another's strategy in social decision making: A transformational analysis. *Journal of Personality and Social Psychology, 55,* 396-409.

McGregor, D. (1960). *The human side of enterprise.* New York: McGraw-Hill.

McGuire, W. J. (1969). The nature of attitudes and attitude change. In G. Lindzey & E. Aronson (Eds.), *The handbook of social psychology* (2nd Ed.). Vol. 3. Reading, MA: Addison-Wesley.

Mechanic, D. & Volkhart, E. H. (1960). Illness behavior and medical diagnosis. *Journal of Health and Human Behavior, 1,* 86-93.

Mehrabian, A. (1971). Nonverbal communication. *Nebraska symposium on motivation, 19,* 107-162.

Menzies, I. (1960). A case-study in the functioning of social systems as a defense against anxiety. *Human Relations, 13,* 95-121.

Merton, R. (1957). *Social theory and social structure.* Glencoe, IL: Free Press.

Miller, J. G. (1965). Living systems: Basic concepts; structure and process: Cross-level hypotheses. *Behavioral Science, 10,* 193-237, 337-411.

Mills, C. W. (1959). *The sociological imagination.* London: Oxford University Press.

Mills, T. M. (1964). *Group transformation.* Englewood Cliffs, N.J.: Prentice Hall.

Mitchell, J. T. (1985). Healing the helper. *Role stressors and supports for emergency workers.* U. S. Department of Health & Human Services Publication, 105-118.

Moos, R. (1976). *The human context: Environmental determinants of behavior.* New York: Wiley.

Moos, R. (1979). Social-ecological perspectives on health. In G. Stone, F. Cohen & N. Adler (Eds.), *Health psychology: A handbook.* San Francisco: Jossey-Bass.

Moos, R. (1980). Specialized living environments for older people: A conceptual framework for evaluation. *Journal of Social Issues, 36,* 75-94.

Moscovici, S. (1985). Social influence and conformity. In G. Lindzey & E. Aronson, (Eds.), *Handbook of social psychology,* (3rd Ed.). 347-412. New York: Random House.

Nadel, S. F. (1957). *The theory of social structure.* Glencoe, Ill.: Free Press.

Nelson, D. L. (1987). Organizational socialization: A stress perspective. *Journal of Occupational Behavior, 8,* 311-324.

Newcomb, T. M. (1961). *The acquaintance process.* New York: Holt, Rinehart & Winston.

Newcomb, T. N. (1958). Attitude development as a function of reference groups: The Bennington study. In E. E. Maccoby, T. M. Newcomb & E. L. Hartley (Eds.), *Readings in social psychology* (3rd Ed.). New York: Holt, Rinehart & Winston.

Newcomb, T. M. (1943). *Personality and social change: Attitude formation in a student community.* New York: Dryden.

Newcomb, T. M., Koenig, K. E., Flacks, R & Warwick, D. P. (1967) *Persistance and change: Bennington College and its students after twenty-five years.* New York: Wiley.

O'Driscoll, M. P. & Evans, R. (1988). Organizational factors and perceptions of climate in three psychiatric units. *Human Relations, 41,* 371-388.

Owan, T. C. O. (Ed.) (1985). *Southeast Asian mental health: Treatment, prevention, services, training and research.* U.S. Department of Health & Human Services Publication.

Patterson, M. (1968). Spatial factors in social interaction. *Human Relations, 21,* 351-361.

Pettigrew, T. F. (1979). The ultimate attribution error: Extending Allport's cognitive analysis of prejudice. *Personality and Social Psychology Bulletin, 5,* 461-476.

Porter, L. W. & Lawler, E. E. (1964). The effects of "tall" versus "flat" organization structures on managerial job satisfaction. *Personnel Psychology, 17,* 135-148.

Rapoport, A. & Chammah, A. M. (1965). *Prisoner's dilemma: A study in conflict and cooperation.* Ann Arbor, MI: University of Michigan Press.

Raven, B. H. & Rubin J. Z. (1976). *Social Psychology: People in groups.* New York: Wiley.

Reinhardt, U. E. (1987). Resource allocation in health care: The allocation of lifestyles to providers. *The Milbank Quarterly, 65,* 153-176.

Relman, A. S. (1980). The new medical-industrial complex. *New England Journal of Medicine, 303,* 963-970.

Ross, L. (1977). The intuitive psychologist and his shortcomings: Distortions in the attribution process. In L. Berkowitz (Ed.), *Advances in experimental social psychology.* Vol. 10, 174-220. New York: Academic Press.

Ruesch, J. & Bateson, G. (1951). *Communication: The social matrix of psychiatry.* New York: Norton.

Runciman, W. G. (1966). *Relative deprivation and social justice: A study of attitudes to social inequality in twentieth-century England.* Berkeley, CA: University of California Press.

Sampson, E. E. (1977). Psychology and the American ideal. *Journal of Personality and Social Psychology, 35,* 767-782.

Sampson, E. E. (1988). The debate on individualism: Indigenous psychologies of the individual and their role in personal and societal functioning. *American Psychologist, 43,* 15-22.

Sarbin, T. R. & Allen, V. L. (1968). Role theory. In G. Lindzey & E. Aronson (Eds.), *Handbook of social psychology* (2nd Ed.) Vol. 1, Reading, MA.: Addison-Wesley.

Schachter, S. (1951). Deviation, rejection, and communication. *Journal of Abnormal and Social Psychology, 46,* 190-207.

Schulman, E. D. (1974). *Intervention in human services.* St. Louis: Mosby.

Schultz, A. (1970-1971). *Collected Papers,* Vols. I-III. The Hague: Martinus Nijhoff.

Schultz, W. C. (1960). *FIRO: A three-dimensional theory of interpersonal behavior.* New York: Holt, Rinehart & Winston.

Scott, W. R. (1981). *Organizations: Rational, natural and open systems.* Englewood Cliffs, N.J.: Prentice-Hall.

Sherif, M. (1935). A study of some social factors in perception. *Archives of Psychology, 27,* no. 187.

Sherif, M. (1966). *Group conflict and cooperation: Their social psychology.* London: Routledge & Kegan Paul.

Sherif, M. & Sherif C. W. (1953). *Groups in harmony and tension.* New York: Harper.

Shumaker, S. A. & Brownell, A. (1985). Social support: New Perspectives in theory, research and intervention. Part II: Interventions and policy. *Journal of Social Issues, 41,* no. 1.

Shweder, R. A. & Bourne, E. (1982). Does the concept of the person vary cross-culturally? In A. J. Marsella & G. White (Eds.), *Cultural concepts of mental health and therapy,* 97-137. Boston: Reidel.

Simmel, G. (1902-1903). The number of members as determining the sociological form of the group. *American Journal of Sociology, 8,* 1-46, 158-196.

Slater, P. E. (1966). *Microcosm.* New York: Wiley.

Smith, S. L. (1951). Communication patterns and the adaptability of task-oriented groups: An experimental study. In D. Lerner & H. Lasswell (Eds.), *The policy sciences: Recent developments in scope and method.* Stanford, Ca.: Stanford University Press.

Sommer, R. (1969). *Personal space,* Englewood Cliffs, N.J.: Prentice-Hall.

Spitz, R. (1945). Hospitalism: An inquiry into the genesis of psychiatric conditions in early childhood. *Psychoanalytic Study of the Child, 1,* 53-74.

Starr, P. (1982). *The social transformation of American medicine.* New York: Basic Books.

Steiger, W. A., Hoffman, F. H., Hansen, V. A., Jr. & Niebuhr, H. (1960). A definition of comprehensive medicine. *Journal of Health and Human Behavior, 1,* 83-85.

Stock, D., Whitman, R. M. & Lieberman, M. A. (1958). The deviant member in therapy groups. *Human Relations, 11,* 341-372.

Stogdill, R. M. (1948). Personal factors associated with leadership. *Journal of Psychology, 25,* 35-71.

Storms, M. D. (1973). Videotape and the attribution process: Reversing actors' and observers' points of view. *Journal of Personality and Social Psychology, 27,* 165-175.

Stouffer, S. A., Suchman, E. A., De Vinney, L. C., Star, S. A. & Williams, R. M., Jr. (1949a). *The American soldier, Vol. 1. Adjustment during army life.* Princeton, N.J.: Princeton University Press.

Stouffer, S. A., Lumsdaine, A. A., Lumsdaine, M. H., Williams, R. M., Jr., Smith, M. B., Janis, I. L., Star, S. A. & Cottrell, L. S. Jr. (1949b). *The American soldier, Vol. 2. Combat and its aftermath.* Princeton, N.J.: Princeton University Press.

Tajfel, H. (1978a). Social categorization, social identity and social comparison. In H. Tajfel (Ed.), *Differentiation between social groups,* 61-76. London: Academic Press.

Tajfel, H. (1978b). *Differentiation between social groups: Studies in the social psychology of intergroup relations.* London: Academic Press.

Tannenbaum, R. & Schmidt, W. H. (1958). How to choose a leadership pattern. *Harvard Business Review, 36,* 95-101.

Taylor, D. M. & Jaggi, V. (1974). Ethnocentrism and causal attribution in a South Indian context. *Journal of Cross-cultural Psychology, 5,* 162-171.

Taylor, D. M. & Moghaddam, F. M. (1987). *Theories of intergroup relations.* New York: Praeger.

Taylor, S. E. & Brown J. D. (1988). Illusion and well-being: A social psychological perspective on mental health. *Psychological Bulletin, 103,* 193-310.

Terhune, K. (1968). Motives situation, and interpersonal conflict within prisoner's dilemma. *Journal of Personality and Social Psychology Monograph Supplement, 8,* 1-24.

Tetlock, P. E. (1985). Integrative complexity of American and Soviet foreign policy rhetoric: A time-series analysis. *Journal of Personality and Social Psychology, 49,* 1565-1585.

Thelen, H. A. (1959). Work-emotionality theory of the group as organism. In S. Koch (Ed.), *Psychology: A study of a science.* Vol. 3. New York: McGraw-Hill.

Thibaut, J. W. & Kelley, H. H. (1959). *The social psychology of groups.* New York: Wiley.

Thoennes, N. A. & Pearson, J. (1985). Predicting outcomes in divorce mediation: The influence of people and process. *Journal of Social Issues, 41,* 115-126.

Tubbs, S. L. (1978). *A systems approach to small group interaction.* Reading, MA: Addison-Wesley.

Tuckman, B. W. (1965). Developmental sequence in small groups. *Psychological Bulletin, 63,* 384-399.

Tversky, A. & Kahneman, D. (1974). Judgment under uncertainty: Heuristics and biases. *Science, 185,* 41-65.

Tylor, T.R. (1987). Procedural justice research. *Social Justice Research, 1,* 41-65.

Vachon, M. L. S. & Stylianos, S. K. (1988). The role of social support in bereavement. *Journal of Social Issues, 44,* 175-190.

Videka, L. (1979). Psychosocial adaptation in a medical self-help group. In M. A. Lieberman, L. Borman & Associates (Eds.), *Self-help groups for coping with crisis,* 362-386. San Francisco, CA: Jossey-Bass.

Watzlawick, P., Beavin, J. H. & Jackson, D. D. (1967). *Pragmatics of Human Communication.* New York: Norton.

Weiss, J. (1952). Crying at the happy ending. *Psychoanalytic Review, 39,* 388.

Wortman, C. B. (1984). Social support and the cancer patient. *Cancer, 15,* 2339-2360.

Yalom, I. D. (1975). *The theory and practice of group psychotherapy.* New York: Basic Books.

Zander, A. F., Cohen, A. R. & Stotland, E. (1957). *Role relations in the mental health professions.* Ann Arbor: Institute for Social Research, University of Michigan.

Zola, I. K. (1966). Culture and symptoms—an analysis of patients' presenting complaints. *American Sociological Review, 31,* 615-630.

Index